The Global Hum
Right to Health

110642351

Dream or possibility?

Théodore H MacDonald PhD, MD, FRSM
Professor (Emeritus) and Associate of Research Institute for Human Rights and
Social Justice
London Metropolitan University
Former Director of Postgraduate Studies in Health, Brunel University
Consultant to the World Health Organization, International Development
Agency and various NGOs in developing countries

Forewords by

Noël A Kinsella

and

John A Gibson

Radcliffe Publishing
Oxford • New York

Radcliffe Publishing Ltd
18 Marcham Road
Abingdon
Oxon OX14 1AA
United Kingdom

www.radcliffe-oxford.com
Electronic catalogue and worldwide online ordering facility.

British Library Cataloguing in Publication Data

A catalogue record for this book is available from the British Library.

ISBN-10 1 84619 201 3
ISBN-13 978 1 84619 201 2

Typeset by Lapiz Digital Services, Chennai, India
Printed and bound by TJI Digital, Padstow, Cornwall, UK

Dedication

This book is gratefully dedicated to the work of

DR MARGARET CHAN

Director General of the World Health Organization

Dr Chan, a Chinese-Canadian physician and medical research worker (communicable diseases), was appointed Director General of WHO on 9 November 2006. She was born in China and came to Canada as a child. Her medical training took place at the University of Western Ontario, from where she graduated in 1976 with the MDCM degree. In 1978 she joined the Public Health Services of the (then) Colony of Hong Kong and by 1994 she became Hong Kong's Director of Health, a post she held for nine years. During that time she organised massive improvements in Public Health, completely reorganising communicable disease surveillance and control, promoting the training corps of public health specialists and established closer local and public health collaboration. She played a prominent role in research on SARS and avian flu. In 1993 she joined the World Health Organization and in 1995 was made Director of Communicable Disease Surveillance for the world body. On her appointment as Director General of WHO, she has stated that her priorities will centre on the health rights of the poorest, especially in Africa, and on women's health rights globally. This author is deeply encouraged by this very positive turn in the fortunes of WHO and wishes her every success in reclaiming ground in the battle for global health equity – ground lost in the last two decades.

Contents

Foreword

The human right to health is an important programmatic right that is recognized in the *International Bill of Human Rights*. Théodore MacDonald provides an analysis of the progress, or lack thereof, in the development of the right to health for all peoples of the world community.

It was John Peters Humphrey, a dear friend and mentor, who would remind us that the United Nations' instruments of human rights clearly articulate the human right to health. We find, for example, in the *Universal Declaration of Human Rights*:

> Article 25:
>
> "1. Everyone has the right to a standard of living adequate for the health and well-being of himself and his family, including food, clothing, housing and medical care and necessary social services, and the right to security in the event of unemployment, sickness, disability, widowhood, old age or other lack of livelihood in circumstances beyond his control."

The lesson taught by Humphrey, who wrote the first draft of the Universal Declaration, known as the Secretariat's Draft, was that this right needed international assistance and co-operation among states if there was to be any substance to the human right to health.

It is, therefore, important to note that the United Nations *International Covenant on Economic, Social and Cultural Rights* reiterates in Article 2 the human right to health and also provides as follows in Article 2:

> Article 2
>
> "1. Each state party to the present Covenant undertakes to take steps, individually and through international assistance and co-operation, especially economic and technical, to the maximum of its available resources, with a view to achieving progressively the full realization of the rights recognized in the present Covenant by all appropriate means, including particularly the adoption of legislative measures."

In this book, MacDonald examines the progress made toward gradually realizing the programmatic right to health and finds that by the mid-1980s advancement was being achieved toward the goal of universal access to primary healthcare. He recalls the forward steps made when Dr Halfdan Mahler was Director General of the World Health Organization and in particular the "Health for All 2000 Campaign". As he observes, the HFA (2000) Campaign set 38 targets to be sought in order to achieve the campaign objectives by the year 2000. But, in fact, few of these were ever achieved. The author argues that this was because, by the late 1980s the influence of WHO had gradually been subsumed by the impact of neoliberal finance in many Third World countries. Since then, indeed, the gap in equity with respect to the human right to health has widened.

The Secretary General of the United Nations, Kofi Annan, tried to get things back on track in 2000 with his initiative known as the "Eight Millennium Development Goals." The target date for achieving these goals is 2020. It is the author's thesis that these objectives constitute a pre-requisite for the achievement of health as a human right. However, he also argues that under present global economic models global equity in health is not possible, and goes on to make a case for an alternative paradigm, expanding on the ideas of International Health Impact Assessments and of Regional Fair Trade Zones.

The passion, conviction and wealth of knowledge of this work's author are evident. His ability as a communicator in conjunction with a tempered expertise held by few enables him to identify, analyze and provide his reflection on the right to health and its relation to global economics. The content and style of the writing reflects MacDonald's impressive experiential background. He has both theoretical and practical roots in multiple fields of inquiry. Having worked as a medical physician in a broad range of the world's poorest nations, he has been witness on a first-hand basis to the inequities against which he has devoted a large portion of his life.

In addition to experiencing on the front lines the difference that primary healthcare can make in the lives of the disadvantaged, Théodore MacDonald is known internationally as a leader in the promotion of the human right to health.

Not only does this work have great heuristic value, it also serves as an example of how the efforts of one remarkable individual can address the concerns of millions.

Noël A Kinsella, PhD, STD
Speaker, Senate of Canada
Chair, Atlantic Human Rights Centre
St. Thomas University, Canada
November 2006

Foreword

> It is to be expected that global inequalities in wealth will, if it persists, lead to global inequalities in access to medical treatment, information and empowerment. (Charlotte Bunch, Executive Director of the Centre for Women's Global Leadership, March 2004)

Today's newspaper (*The Age*: Saturday 11 November 2006) echoes the broader themes of global inequality concerning the parlous and preventable state of the health of millions in the Third World and the injurious effect of neoliberal economic policies in world trade and global finance which resonate throughout Professor MacDonald's book. The following items are quoted:

> A report to the US Congress reveals the true extent of the carnage in Iraq.

> US Ambassador to the UN John Bolton's position is under threat following the overwhelming mid-term Democratic election victory.

> UNDP calls for clean water to save the lives of nearly 2 million children a year who die because of polluted water supplies and a want of proper sanitation, while the world's poor often pay more for their water than people in the US and Britain. In Africa's largest slum (Kibera, on the outskirts of Nairobi) where between half a million to a million people live in abject poverty, contaminated water and lack of sanitation produce constant illness.

> A Chinese bureaucrat Dr Margaret Chan (*see* Endnote) is appointed head of WHO and concerns are raised in the light of the past secrecy of the PRC authorities in dealing with the SARS epidemic as to whether she will be able to stand up to her own country when it matters.

> A lead article explores the power shift in the US while noting that all the global challenges to world peace and stability remain: the threat and consequences of global warming, the effects of globalisation, world trade arrangements, the future of the UN, the global battle against AIDS and poverty.

All these subjects form important threads in Professor MacDonald's analysis and emphasise the contemporary relevance and importance of his work.

The author draws upon his own experience as a medical doctor and mathematician who has lived and worked in a broad range of the world's poorest nations, and provides us with a human rights-based framework with which to understand the true state of the health of billions in the world and the historical and geo-political reasons for this. He advances a multi-faceted argument that the UN Charter asserted the aim of establishing global equity in human rights and one of those rights was 'universal access to primary healthcare', yet the equity gap with respect to this has been steadily widening – not the reverse. He shows empirically how health is so integral to world peace, security and stability and the alleviation of poverty and that disease is a major obstacle to social progress and equity.

Importantly, he offers practical suggestions and gives examples of how this situation can be turned around and identifies the options in many different fields that need to be explored to achieve this goal. It is absolutely vital to the future of the world, he says, that the Millennium Development Goals be achieved as a necessary pre-requisite to the realisation of the right to primary healthcare. Given the wealth of the developed world and the potential energies and abilities of the less developed world, there is no reason to doubt that these goals are achievable. There is no lack of material resources; what is needed is the will. Present failure can only be overcome by nations transcending national interests in response to global needs and the neoliberal agenda and interests of transnational corporations must be reined in through transnational control of trade (using for example Regional Fair Trading Zones). He is optimistic about the US playing a constructive leading role in finding a means of globalisation consistent with human rights. He envisages, not without good reason, the possibility of Chinese financial hegemony. A cohesive UN which is able to oversee and implement the desired changes in global relationships and be able to fulfil its peace-keeping mandate, he views as essential.

As just one example of inter-relationships having multi-dimensional effects, Professor MacDonald emphasises the centrality of the need for equitable distribution of water resources within and between states as a pivotal factor in improving world health, combating disease and for reducing the incidence of human conflict which itself produces a whole range of highly destructive direct and indirect environmental and health consequences.

There are a number of occasions throughout the book where the author provides a clear and concise definitional explanation of important terms or concepts which greatly inform a lay reader like myself. His arguments are invariably backed up by hard empirical data drawn from a range of authoritative sources.

Some of his themes directly relate to my areas of concern – such as the proliferation of trafficking in women and children and the continuing hideous abuse of female genital mutilation – itself giving rise to refugee status (see *Secretary of State for the Home Department (Respondent) v. K (FC) (Appellant) Fornah (FC) (Appellant) v. Secretary of State for the Home Department (Respondent)* [2006] UKHL 46) as well as the broader issue of movements of peoples for reasons related to the Refugees Convention or for broader humanitarian reasons. While the necessity for a legal definition of a term like 'refugee' must be recognised, his analysis demonstrates again the difficulty of sometimes distinguishing in both legal and humanitarian terms between those who leave their homes because of Convention-related persecution and those forced to move because of conflict or poverty in circumstances where lack of water and/or food is causing severe health deficits.

My first meeting with Theo MacDonald was at a conference in August 2005 convened by RMIT University of Melbourne in conjunction with UNDP on 'Pathways to Reconciliation and Global Human Rights' in Sarajevo in Bosnia-Herzegovina, focusing with great poignancy on that country particularly. I, as a lawyer specialising in refugee law with a human rights focus, and he, as a health specialist and polymath, were joined by a range of experts from a number of different countries in the practical and moral issues of post-conflict reconciliation. His presence at that conference, as this book shows, was an indication of the extraordinary breadth of his knowledge and interests. In a world of increasing specialisation and narrow academic focus it was a pleasure for me to be confronted and challenged, as well as informed, on many different conceptual and thematic levels by Professor MacDonald's work.

The Global Human Right to Health: dream or possibility? significantly adds to the understanding of health as a fundamental human right, the content of that right and what must be done to ensure that it can become a reality for the millions who presently lack even an acceptable standard of primary healthcare. The reader is left with a clear message; unless we evaluate alternatives to existing structures to bring about qualitative change in health outcomes in the developing world, environmental disaster fuelled by war and international chaos is our probable destiny.

I am honoured to have been asked to write this foreword and enthusiastically recommend it to anyone with an interest in the future of mankind.

John A Gibson
Barrister
President of the Refugee Council of Australia
Remembrance Day, 11 November 2006

Endnote: *See* the Author's Dedication

Preface

If health is a basic human right, as indicated both in the UN Charter and in the UN Declaration of Human Rights, then so obviously is primary healthcare (PHC). It was PHC that Dr Halfdan Mahler, the Danish Director General of the World Health Organization (WHO), set out to make universal during his tenure of office in the 1980s. He called the enterprise Health For All 2000 (HFA 2000).

As the author explains, that campaign fizzled out under pressure from neoliberal forces after he had left office, and the global inequities in health (and certainly in PHC) are now very great indeed. The UN finds itself divided on the issue because, while it obviously supports its original Charter, and while it is true that the WHO is a UN agency, it is also true that the World Bank, the International Monetary Fund (IMF) and the World Trade Organization (WTO) are also UN agencies. As a result, the WHO has become progressively less able to promote HFA.

Under the leadership of Kofi Annan, the UN convened a council in 2000 and promulgated eight Millennium Development Goals (MDGs), to be achieved by 2015, in an attempt to steer the world body back into arbitrating global equity in health and other human rights. In analysing these MDGs, this author realised that the global human right to health cannot even begin to be realised unless the eight MDGs are achieved – and in less than ten years!

This book is therefore based on a close scrutiny of these eight MDGs and our progress towards meeting them, and the chapters generally deal with them systematically. The only real exceptions to this are Chapters 5 and 15.

In Chapter 5 the author provides a reader-friendly explanation of how the Gini coefficient works and how to calculate it. The Gini coefficient is now widely used in discourses comparing the average income of one country with that of another, and comparing individual incomes within a single country. Gini scores are routinely quoted in government documents and research papers dealing with human rights issues. Thus unless the reader has a reasonable grasp of the central ideas, they will have difficulty in understanding policy statements, etc., based on such findings.

Chapter 15, after summing up the arguments to that point, tackles the issue of alternatives to neoliberalism as a global finance and trade mechanism. The author does this on the basis that, unless we evaluate such alternatives, the human right to equity in health must remain a mere dream, as the world hurtles towards environmental disaster fuelled by war and international chaos.

Théodore H MacDonald
Littlehampton
England
November 2006

Acknowledgements

It is always difficult to write an acknowledgement for a book of this complexity, which has drawn on the resources of so many agencies, experts and colleagues in the field. Many of these must go unacknowledged in the interest of space. However, in relation to the immediate production and processing of the manuscript of this book, I must mention the following:

Mrs Betty Maund and Ms Beth Archer word-processed the manuscript from my handwritten version. Their skill, patience and dexterity in coping with the irascibilities of computer technology were an inspiration. My son, Matthew, and my wife, Chris, were also hugely helpful in this regard. I am also immensely indebted to Chris for her forbearance during the domestic chaos that the writing of a book inevitably entails.

The publishers, as always, have made this book possible as a result of their ready professionalism and editorial skills. In this context, I wish to thank the commissioning editor, Gillian Nineham, the project manager, Paula Jales, and the editorial assistant, Lisa Abbott.

Any errors or imperfections in this book are the author's alone.

Chapter 1

Human rights: the UN's mandate

The Millennium Development Goals

The expression 'human rights' only became widely used once it was enshrined in the United Nations (UN) Charter back in 1945. And in those first heady days, although the challenges facing human rights were recognised as great, at least the mechanisms seemed to have been put in place to promote and sustain human rights globally. All of this was cause for optimism indeed. But in the intervening years much of the hope, commitment and idealism drained away, as the UN seemed to lose power and influence and itself fall prey to infighting and the intrusion of influences designed to protect and further the interests of developed nations at increasing expense to less developed nations.

Much of the UN's effectiveness in defending global human rights naturally depends on its Secretary General, and we are currently fortunate in having Kofi Annan as a leader who has been insistent on the primacy of human rights and equally vehement in declaring that a precursor to global human rights has to be the eradiation of poverty.

In September 2000, at the United Nations Millennium Summit in Geneva, a list of eight 'Millennium Development Goals' (MDGs) was finally agreed by 189 national heads of state (subsequently increased to 190). The Summit also agreed that the year 2015 should be the deadline for the fulfilment of these goals. The MDGs, which are intended to be 'universal' – that is, to apply globally and without exception – are as follows:

1 the eradication of extreme poverty
2 the achievement of universal primary education
3 the promotion of gender equality and the empowerment of women
4 the reduction of child mortality
5 the improvement of maternal health
6 the combating of HIV/AIDS, malaria, tuberculosis and other diseases
7 the establishment of environmental sustainability worldwide
8 the development of a global partnership for development.

At one of the subsequent meetings to consider progress towards the MDGs (in New York on 9 September 2005), Kofi Annan made the following statement:

> We will have time to reach the Millennium Development Goals – worldwide and in most, or even all, individual countries – but only if we break with business as usual action across the entire decade between now and the deadline. It takes time to train the teachers, nurses and engineers, to build the roads, schools and hospitals, and to grow the small and large businesses able to create the jobs and income needed. So we must start now. And we must more than double global development assistance over the next few years. Nothing less will help to achieve the Goals.[1]

Why the MDGs are a minimal basis

It will be readily apparent to the reader that these goals are a minimum basis for creating a global context for equity in health and other human rights. If we achieve the MDGs, then the human rights defined in the UN Charter will be a possibility. If we do not, then the idea of global human rights must remain a dream. It is quite simple.

Already we can see plenty of room for manoeuvre, prevarication and delay by people anxious to avoid compliance. For instance, can we secure agreement on what is meant by 'extreme poverty' in MDG 1? How much 'promotion' should there be in MDG 3 and how will it be assessed? By how much would child mortality need to be reduced in order to satisfy MDG 4? And so on. However, if the relevant committees were satisfied by the target date that the goals had been met, we would be in a position to create transnational mechanisms for establishing and sustaining global equity in human rights.

Yet achievement of these goals is already threatened by two main factors:

1 unacceptable delays in implementation on the ground
2 resistance to the MDGs in the developed world.

Thus although some significant progress is being made towards meeting some of the targets in some of the affected countries, in many other parts of the world progress has been slow, patchy or even non-existent. This is due to a large number of often local factors which will be discussed in greater detail in subsequent chapters. To assist local implementation of the goals, a series of 18 targets was also drawn up so that the international community could recognise whether appropriate progress was being made in particular regions, and give appropriate advice if required. Factors that impede such delicate arrangements include wars, internal corruption and, above all, the vastly increasing impact of transnational corporate interests protecting their own investments in the developing world. For instance, in sub-Saharan Africa, the number of people living in extreme poverty is greater now (in 2006) than it was in 1990.

Much more worrying still is resistance to the MDGs by the developed nations at the highest levels. Much of the commentary in this book deals with this issue, as it is a very real threat. For now, suffice it to say that the USA has led the developed world in financial and military terms since the 1940s, and it was under its aegis that such organisations as the World Bank, the International Monetary Fund (IMF) and the World Trade Organization (WTO) came into being. Although they fulfil their global responsibilities as UN agencies, this book shows quite clearly that these and similar bodies are also assiduous in promoting and protecting US corporate interests. Likewise, US governmental representatives to the UN are serving two masters – their national interests and the global aims of the UN.

As the author points out throughout this book, this does not vitiate the role of the USA in the UN. The USA is a complex and energetic civilisation with much to offer in the realm of human rights. The less developed countries (LDCs) and progressive international thinking have valuable support in the USA. However, in 2005 President Bush appointed John Bolten as 'acting' US Ambassador to the UN while awaiting formal approval of the appointment some time after the US mid-term elections. However, it now appears that

President Bush may not get his way on this due to those election results, and Mr Bolten will not be given the post. In the meantime though, John Bolten has seemed intent on representing US corporate interests in the LDCs which run counter to the MDGs in some respects. These issues are dealt with in greater detail in subsequent chapters, but Bolten has been hostile to both the present administration of the UN and its MDGs.

It is important to mention this here, because Bolten's impact at the 2005 MDG summit in New York does not augur well for the prospects of either the UN itself or its MDGs. A month prior to that summit, in August 2005, John Bolten dropped his first bombshell when he submitted to the committee that was drawing up the 2005 UN Report a list of 750 alterations which he wanted made to the text – itself only 39 pages long! Outstanding among his many scathing criticisms was that he wanted all 14 references to the MDGs to be deleted. The goals that Bolten wanted removed included reducing by half the number of people living on less than US$ 1.00 per day by 2015. That number, by the way, was 1.3 billion people in 2005. It is true that, although the USA had not signed the agreement, people had been under the impression that the Bush administration would not actually oppose them – until John Bolten came on board to do the President's will.

This does not bode well for the project as far as global human rights are concerned. In this author's view, we must be both informed about the UN and ready to defend it as an institution. Only from such a position of security can it confidently deliver on its mandate to, for instance, order the recruitment of international peace-keeping forces in conflict zones, work effectively to prevent such evils as the trafficking of women and children for prostitution, organise international control of transnational corporations and their cartels, and so on.

As the reader makes their way through this book, they should keep in mind the unique aspects of the MDGs, and their cruciality in establishing global equity in human rights. Some of their unique features include, or strongly imply, the following.

- The MDGs constitute a compact between the world's major economic players and those in less developed nations. While the latter are called upon to improve policies and governance, and to increase accountability to their own citizens, wealthy developed countries are pledged to provide resources when called upon by the UN to do so. Because commitment to achieving the goals comes from the highest political levels this means that, for the first time in history, governments are committed individually to the goals as part of their national policy programmes. And this must include the trade and finance ministers from the powerful nations. These individuals, both figuratively and literally, hold the world's purse-strings. In the same way, such major international financial institutions as the World Bank, the IMF, regional development banks and the WTO have explicitly agreed to be accountable for achieving the goals.
- Never before has there been so much prosperity. For instance, the hundreds of billions of dollars that are being squandered on military adventures everywhere from the Republic of the Congo to Iraq have served to put things in perspective – and to remind us that we would need no more than US$ 50 billion

each year to meet the goals. This could be mediated as aid. In 2003, about US$ 900 billion were invested in arms by governments. Consider also that the wealthy nations grant agricultural subsidies of about US$ 300 billion per year. At a purely financial level, then, we are not talking about much money, but about huge shifts in mindset.

- It is essential that progress in meeting the MDGs is monitored. That is, the goals cannot merely be idealistic statements. Precise monitoring mechanisms have been put in place by insisting that each government reports at specific time intervals on the millennium goals, and that the Secretary General of the UN reports once a year to the General Assembly of the UN, thus putting pressure on governments to maintain the highest standards. More than 60 such country reports (out of 190) have already been produced at the national level.

- There are no insurmountable obstacles to achieving these goals, only psychological ones. That does not make them easy to overcome, but any failure to meet the goals can never be blamed on lack of material resources. As this author argues in the Preface and throughout this book, the goals may be called 'Millennium' Development Goals, but they are more than that – they are 'Minimum' Development Goals. The bar cannot drop below this standard, and the MDGs constitute minimal bases required to finally achieve global equity in human rights.

To quote Millennium Campaign News:[2]

> The Goals cover the range of key development issues and are rooted in a human rights framework. Freedom, equality, solidarity, tolerance, respect for nature and shared responsibility are at the heart of the Millennium Declaration. The eight Goals are by nature inter-linked. Success or failure on any one Goal will affect efforts to achieve all the others. And at their core, the Goals are about people's lives. There is often a tendency to measure success in the aggregate – for example, how many more children are in school this year, and how many more women survived childbirth in 2003. This can give us a sense of how well or badly we are doing, but the most important question to bear in mind is this: how have people's real lives been affected by our efforts to achieve the Goals? It is important to know how each individual, each region and each sub-region is affected as we strive to reach the Goals by 2015.

Given the level of prosperity in the First World now in 2006, we can easily pay for all the MDGs, and we also have at our disposal all of the technical expertise necessary to set up any infrastructure contingent upon them, such as water reticulation systems, etc. However, if we let things continue to slide as they are doing, the MDGs will not be realised and therefore neither will the UN Charter provisions for human rights.

As stated in the Preface, this author's argument is that the real and overriding issue is to find an alternative method of global finance to that espoused by neoliberal economic theory. There are alternatives to consider, as discussed in the final chapter.

References

1 Annan K. *Statement by UN Secretary General Kofi A Annan at the Millennium Development Goals Progress Meeting*, UN, New York, 9 September 2005; www.un.org/millenniumgoals/index.asp (accessed 2 June 2006).
2 Millennium Campaign (2005) *Voices Against Poverty*; www.millenniumcampaign.org/site/pp.asp?c-grKVLZNLEs (accessed 2 June 2006).

Chapter 2

A bird's-eye view of global finance and human rights

The players

The reader is about to enter into a discussion about issues that in some respects resemble a Russian novel in its complexity of plots, counterplots and characters. Of course, in this context not all of the 'characters' are individual people, but large institutions. Some are household words – the UN, UNESCO, UNICEF and WHO – and of these some are known by name but not widely understood. These and similar institutions operate through various procedures which tend to go under the sobriquet of esoteric acronyms (SAPs, TRIPS, GATT, etc.). Therefore, let us first introduce a few of these pivotal entities.

The United Nations (UN) and its Charter

During the early months of 1945, as World War Two was drawing to a close, representatives of 50 nations met in San Francisco to establish the UN. As the reader probably knows, the UN was established as an international organisation to promote international security, cooperation and peace. The impetus for its establishment was to prevent the horror of internecine strife, from which the world was just emerging, and to produce a global body that would be more effective than the pre-war League of Nations. Its headquarters is now in New York.

Fundamental to world peace is, of course, the concept of human rights, and this was the focus of the San Francisco meeting referred to above. At that conference the 50 nations adopted the UN Charter, a document which sets forth the UN's goals, functions and responsibilities. Human rights have priority in the Charter right from the start. Article 1 of the Charter states that one of the aims of the UN is to achieve international cooperation in 'promoting and encouraging respect for human rights and for fundamental freedoms for all without distinction as to the race, sex, language or religion.'

However, the goals of Article 1 of the Charter are general ones, and we needed unambiguous definitions of specific human rights before we could proceed. To that end the Commission on Human Rights was established, and it was charged with creating the International Bill of Human Rights. The latter consists of the Universal Declaration of Human Rights (UDHR), the International Covenant on Civil and Political Rights (and its Protocol) and the International Covenant on Economics, Social and Cultural Rights.

The UDHR was the first off the planning table, and its role was to define the 'basic human rights' to which we refer in this book and to which all individuals anywhere in the world are entitled. Unfortunately, however, a 'declaration' is not legally binding. For the rights defined by it to have full legal force, they must be incorporated into 'conventions' (sometimes referred to as *treaties* or *covenants*), and it is these which set out the international norms and standards. Wherever a government signs (ratifies) such a convention, that nation becomes legally required to uphold these standards.

In this way, the UDHR spawned two covenants critical to our discussion, namely the International Covenant on Civil and Political Rights (ICCPR), along with its Protocol, and the International Covenant on Economics, Social and Cultural Rights (ICESCR). These, like every other such covenant, establish procedures for monitoring and reporting how signatories to the conventions concerned are complying with it. Article 1 in the ICCPR established a Human Rights Committee of 18 independent experts whose role was to examine the remitting reports. It is also in the remit of the committee to provide a complaints procedure through which individuals or groups who have a grievance against their government can be heard at an international forum.

Whenever a UN member ratifies such a convention, it not only agrees to abide by the provisions of the convention, but also consents to be monitored. Most of the violations of human rights discussed in this book are exacerbated by ambivalence on the issue of international monitoring. The UN member must also agree to alter its laws to conform to the convention, and to report such changes at regular intervals. Relevant sections of these reports are also forwarded to other UN-affiliated intergovernmental organisations, such as the World Health Organization (WHO) and the International Labour Organization (ILO), for their analysis and recommendations.

How conventions are formed

Obviously, moving a human rights idea on to an internationally legally binding convention is no quick or simple matter, and the avoidance of such challenges was one of the reasons that rendered the old League of Nations ineffectual. The process is a lengthy and tortuous one involving consensus and trust building and the nitty-gritty of practical policies at both national and international levels. The procedure can be briefly summarised as follows.[1]

1   *Drafting.* The proposed convention is drafted by various interested groups. The UN General Assembly commissions these groups, which consist of representatives of UN member states as well as people representing both existing intergovernmental and non-governmental organisations (NGOs).
2   *Adoption by the UN.* The proposal is then adopted or rejected by a vote of the UN General Assembly.
3   *Signing by Member States.* Whenever a member state signs the proposed convention, they are indicating that they have started the process required by their government for formal notification. By signing they also agree to refrain from acts that would be contrary to the objectives of the convention.
4   *Ratification.* When a member state ratifies a convention, it obviously agrees to comply with its provisions and obligations. To this end it assumes the responsibility to ensure that national legislation does not conflict with the convention, while at the same time indicating its reservations about any specific articles of the convention. As we shall see, this can lead to months or years of delay, during which much needless suffering of innocent people can occur.
5   *Entering into force.* A convention comes into effect when a certain number of member states have ratified it. For example, the ICCPR and the ICESCR were

originally adopted in 1966, but it was not until a decade later, in 1976, that the specified number of member states (35 at the time) ratified them.

This process may strike the reader as rather protracted, but in fact it rarely moves as smoothly as indicated above. A major obstruction occurs because of variations in legislation within nations. For instance, in the USA the process towards ratification begins when the President endorses the document by signing it. It is then submitted to the Senate, along with any administrative recommendations. The Senate Foreign Relations Committee first considers the convention, conducting hearings to monitor public reaction. The Foreign Relations Committee may then recommend the convention to the Senate, possibly with reservations or qualifications. Such reservations are often based on the need to enact new legislation in order to conform to a convention. However, the federal system of the US government gives individual states, not the national government, the right to make law in many areas, such as criminal and family law. Next the full Senate considers the convention. Finally, if the Senate approves the convention, the President formally notifies the UN that the USA has ratified and thus become a state party to the convention.

The Convention on the Rights of the Child provides an example of the evolution of a UN Convention. In 1959, a working group drafted the Declaration on the Rights of the Child, which consisted of 10 principles setting forth basic rights to which all children should be entitled.

The Rights of the Child: declaration to conventions

Pivotal as a major concern in this book is the impact on the health rights of children. The basic principles were easily agreed upon by member states, and agreement on the declaration was not difficult to secure. However, it was in codifying these principles into a convention that problems arose. A summary of the whole convoluted process is highly instructive and provides a basis on which improvements in securing global rights might well be initiated.

The formal drafting process lasted for nine years, during which representatives of governments, intergovernmental agencies such as UNICEF and UNESCO, and non-governmental organisations (NGOs) such as Save the Children and the International Red Cross, worked together to create consensus on the language to be used in the Convention.

The resulting Convention on the Rights of the Child (Children's Convention) contains 54 articles that can be divided into three general categories:

1 protection – covering specific issues, such as abuse, neglect and exploitation
2 provision – addressing a child's particular needs, such as education and healthcare
3 participation – acknowledging a child's growing capacity to make decisions and play a part in society.

The Children's Convention was adopted by the General Assembly in 1989, and was immediately signed and ratified by more nations and in a shorter period of time than any other UN convention. As a result, the Children's Convention entered into force shortly thereafter, in 1990. Furthermore, the total number of member states that have ratified the Children's Convention has surpassed that for all other conventions.

As of December 1998, only two member states have not ratified the Children's Convention, namely Somalia and the USA. It goes without saying that if the most powerful and wealthy nation on Earth cannot ratify something as basic as the Convention on the Rights of the Child, we are facing an uphill struggle if we are to truly make 'primary healthcare' a basic human right.

In the 58 years from 1948 to 2006, the UDHR has produced 20 human rights conventions. Many have already come into force, while the others are still in the process of ratification. One in particular that has not yet even been drafted is a convention on the rights of indigenous people. Indeed, as will be discussed later in this text, the *British Medical Journal* has considered this crucial topic in recent issues, not only with respect to indigenous people living in First World nations such as Australia or the USA, but also with respect to indigenous people in India, African nations, South America, etc.

The World Health Organization

The WHO was formally established on 7 April 1948 as the UN's specialist agency for health. As stated in its Constitution,[2] the objective of the WHO is the attainment by all peoples of the highest possible level of health. The constitution then goes on to define health as a 'state of complete physical, mental and social well-being and not merely the absence of disease or infirmity.' This definition obviously casts its remit very broadly indeed, for if we are not speaking only of the 'absence of disease', we are referring to much more than clinical or biomedical criteria. Indeed, we are referring to health promotion.[3] This in turn must involve – at the very least – primary healthcare (PHC). PHC is defined in slightly different ways by different health agencies. For instance, within biomedical circles, it is just the first rung of a three-rung hierarchy consisting of primary healthcare (PHC), secondary healthcare (SHC) and tertiary healthcare (THC), where PHC refers to access to a general medical practitioner and possibly a nurse or health visitor, SCH refers to clinical facilities and more diagnostic tests (e.g. X-ray) and THC refers to the most esoteric levels of medical technology, specialist surgery, etc. However, this is not what the WHO meant by PHC, nor was it what the UN Charter had in mind when it referred to PHC as a 'human right.'[4] Not only does PHC have a wider remit than the 'operational' definition given above (because it includes access to dentistry and to pharmaceuticals), but also it embraces all of the social contexts that enhance health.

The working definition of PHC in this context was elaborated by the WHO in 1978 in its now famous Alma Ata Declaration.[5] In general, it was held to be a strategy that not only responds equitably, appropriately and effectively to clinical healthcare needs, but also deals comprehensively with social, economic and political causes and consequences of poor health. At a meeting of the International Peoples' Health University (IPHU) in Cuenca, Ecuador in July 2005, PHC was defined by David Sanders[6] as including the following:

1 It must be applicable universally and converge on the basis of need only.
2 It must be comprehensive in that it emphasises disease prevention *and* health promotion.
3 It must embrace both individual and community involvement and inculcate responsibility for maintaining health.

4 It must be intersectorial, involving cooperation between all of the relevant agencies (education, law enforcement, medical, etc.).

5 It must include access on the basis of need alone to all available medical or diagnostic technology that resources allow.

The WHO has continued to play a key role in promoting the need to make PHC realisable as a 'human right', and indeed in this it has been perfectly consistent with the UN Charter. However, since 1988 it has been running into difficulties. As the author pointed out in 2005,[7] the original guiding WHO principles of PHC as a basic human right have been increasingly sidelined as a result of financial globalisation under such mechanisms as the International Monetary Fund, Structural Adjustment Policies and World Trade Organization imposition of policies under the General Agreement on Trade in Services. Instead of health being regarded as a basic human right (as it is in the UN Charter), it has become more and more of a 'desideratum if it can be afforded.'

This can be seen by looking at the policies and priorities of various Director Generals of the WHO from 1948 until the present day.

Director Generals of the WHO

As of 2006, there had been six Director Generals of the WHO, each bringing their own dynamic approach to the post. As the reader will appreciate, they have all been remarkable people and each has been dedicated in his or her own way to the deepest interests of the WHO's initial commitments, but one can see from the following brief accounts how the emphasis has gradually shifted from PHC as a basic human right to the establishment of a coherent financial basis for PHC. Thus Dr B Chrisholm (Canada) saw the role of the WHO to be that of a global agency for addressing the serious traumas incurred by World War Two and the huge backlog of disease and depredation that conflict had left in its wake. One of the really critical issues that he addressed during his tenure was the organisation of immunisation programmes in a world in which much of the healthcare infrastructure had been destroyed. By the time Dr MG Candau (Brazil) assumed the Director Generalship in 1953, many of the purely clinical and specific illness-directed issues were being addressed. He pushed the boundaries further, and confidentially stated that smallpox would be eliminated worldwide in the foreseeable future. He also averred, and many agreed with him, that poliomyelitis would likewise soon be a bad memory of the past. More than 50 years later, it is still regrettably with us, and it can be agreed that at least some of the responsibility for that delay can be laid at the door of the gradual loss of universal PHC as a priority objective.

In 1973, Dr Halfdan Mahler (Denmark) assumed the mantle of Director General. He was tireless throughout his tenure, which ended in 1988, in aggressively pursuing global PHC as a priority. Indeed, he organised committees to draw up strategies for creating 'Health for All' by the year 2000. His HFA policies even formed the basis of the now famous 'Healthy Cities' programmes, the first of which gave rise to the 'Ottawa Charter 1986',[8] a major influential vehicle in popularising the health promotion ideas of Marc Lalonde.[9] His term of office represented the high point in the self-confidence of the WHO, in this author's view, in that it was heading towards the realisation of PHC as a global goal.

Dr H Nakajima (Japan), whose tenure ran from 1988 to 1989, was concerned that the WHO's goals should be tied in more closely with the increasing dominance of neoliberal financial orthodoxies, with its emphasis on open markets and free trade worldwide. He also came to the post with a sound research background in HIV/AIDS, and set about applying this expertise in elaborating policies to confront the issue, and he emphasised the importance of widespread educational campaigns about it.

A strong political insight became evident in the leadership of the WHO when the eminent Norwegian physician and public health specialist, Dr GH Brundtland, became its Director General in 1997.[10] Her academic background had prepared her admirably for work in public health (she had done so well in her basic medical studies in Oslo that she won a postgraduate fellowship to do a research degree in public health at Harvard). However, the cut and thrust of politics had formed an important part of her upbringing. Her father, himself an eminent medical man, had been Minister of Defence in Norway's Labour Party, and she readily joined the youth wing of that organisation at the age of seven! She became adept at political debate at the family dinner table, and she was given every encouragement to believe that women had a crucial role to play in both medical and political leadership.

After she had been in office for three months as Director General, Brundtland was quoted as saying, 'There is a very close connection between being a doctor and a politician. The doctor tries to prevent illness and then tries to treat it if it comes. The politician tries to do the same, but with regard to society instead of individual patients.' Her first official initiative at the WHO completely altered its basic structure, dividing it into nine separate clusters of programmes. Paramount among her achievements were two programmes aimed at the eradication of non-communicable disease, such as malaria, and the first ever national tobacco-free initiative, sponsoring an intensive research programme on developing an HIV/AIDS vaccine, and a global 'Stop TB Project.' She also turned her attention towards what she called 'sustainable health financial systems.' It was probably this, in the present author's view, that gave rise to the idea of PHC being contingent on an integrated system of global finance, rather than being a 'basic human right.' That, of course, was not how Brundtland saw it at the time, and indeed she is quoted as saying 'WHO has to be the vocal force to drive home the message that poverty remains the biggest source of ill health, and it thus engenders succeeding generations of poverty.'[11] She further emphasised the importance of finance in fighting disease when she said on 10 November 1998, in a speech to the Permanent Mission of the UN in Geneva, 'We need to present the evidence and to develop the language to demonstrate that the right investments in health to all − but especially to women and children − mean first of all to develop a strong economy.'[12]

The last-but-one Director General of the WHO was the Korean physician and medical researcher Dr Lee Jong-Wook. He assumed this post on 21 May 2003, but regrettably died (following brain surgery) while still in office, on 22 May 2006, barely three years later. His had been an ideal Director Generalship in many respects, not least because he was equally fluent in Korean, Japanese, French and English. Amazingly broadly educated, he could converse equally readily about English romantic poetry, medicine or particle physics![13]

After Dr Lee, Dr Anders Norström was made Acting Director on 11 October, 2006. But on 9 November, Dr Margaret Chan was appointed the new Director General of WHO, *see* Dedication page for details.

During Dr Lee's time in office, he was confronted with the severe acute respiratory syndrome (SARS) outbreak and then with avian flu. He addressed both issues energetically and pragmatically. He quickly realised that a major impediment to the WHO's global effectiveness was the need for a system of international communication in much of the Third World, and within his first year in office he had satellite dishes installed in country offices that had previously been inaccessible by phone. He also presided over difficult reforms and financial cuts to ensure that more of the WHO budget could be directed towards areas of greatest need. It was he who launched the famous '3 by 5' campaign which aimed to get life-saving antiretroviral drugs (ARVs) to 3 million people in the LDCs by the end of 2005. He intended this to be the first step towards the goal of making HIV/AIDS prevention and treatment universally accessible as a human right for all who need it.

Ultimately this bold initiative failed, but by the end of 2005, 1.3 million people were being equipped with the necessary ARVs, and because of this many commentators regard the initiative as having been successful in its own right. It has certainly resulted in a much better global appreciation of the problem, and has brought about a huge increase in the establishment of clinics and of sex-education centres. Above all, it has finally made the issue of HIV/AIDS a respectable topic of conversation and debate in societies where, until now, it was regarded as taboo. At the G8 summit in 2005, it was agreed that the project should continue, with a target of universal access set for 2010. In a speech which Dr Lee Jong-Wook was due to give to the World Health Assembly on the day he died, he wrote, 'There can be no comfort level in the fight against HIV. We must go on!'[14]

He had already established himself as a global figure in public health long before he assumed the leadership of the WHO. In 1970 he had become Head of Polio Eradication in the Western Pacific, where he oversaw a reduction in the number of cases from 6,000 to 700 within three years. Four years later he became Director of the WHO Vaccines and Immigration Programme in Geneva. There his reputation in global public health grew, and he started initiatives to cooperate with the pharmaceutical industry in the development of new vaccines. By 1998 he had become a serious policy adviser to Gro Brundtland in elaborating financial reforms in the WHO's allocation of resources, and he was appointed Director of the WHO TB Department in 2000. In that post he established the WHO's first large-scale public/private health initiative, namely the Global Partnership to Stop TB, throwing his energies into simultaneous sub-programmes to get TB drug treatment to patients in the poorest countries.

Probably his final initiative before his untimely death was his appointment of Dr Arati Kochi as Director of the WHO Malaria Department in 2002, with an explicit demand to shake things up. Dr Kochi, with Dr Lee's encouragement, began by issuing warnings to the major pharmaceutical companies to market the new artemisinin antimalarial drugs only in combination with older prophylactics, in order to prevent resistance developing and to increase their potency.[15]

In this brief account of the contributions of the Director Generals of the WHO from 1948 until 2006, the author has attempted to show how the initial emphasis on the ideology about global PHC has gradually changed. Moreover, these changes have not come about through any dereliction of duty or commitment by the leadership in the WHO itself, but because of the parallel growth and development of mechanisms for ensuring the global imposition of neoliberal financial policies. The WHO has responded to this imposition of financial power, compelled to do so by the realities of the situation, and without the selfless commitment of the leadership over the years to the defence and enhancement of PHC, public health worldwide would be in an even worse situation than it is in now. What this author's argument will ultimately suggest is that, unless we elaborate alternative and robust systems of globalised finance, the WHO will never be able to establish PHC as a realistic basis for universal human rights. The rest of this chapter, then, will briefly introduce the other key figures and the means by which they are sustaining neoliberal financial orthodoxies on a global scale.

The primary agencies of concern to us in this context are the World Bank, the International Monetary Fund (IMF) and the World Trade Organization (WTO). Each of these bodies is linked to a huge array of means for accomplishing its objectives. The principal ones are structural adjustment policies (SAPs), General Agreement on Tariffs and Trade (GATT) and General Agreement on Trade in Services (GATS). In this chapter, the author will give a brief account of these agencies, showing how they interrelate. Chapter 3 will give a much more complete account, and it forms the basis for an analysis of their often negative impact on health and other human rights, even in the developed world, but especially in the less developed countries.

The World Bank and the International Monetary Fund

The World Bank and the IMF are sometimes referred to as 'twin sisters', because they both emerged from the Bretton Woods Conference that was convened in July 1944. It must be remembered, of course, that this was just as the most calamitous war ever experienced on Earth was drawing to a close. The pleasant New Hampshire town of Bretton Woods seemed like an ideally idyllic place for world leaders to calmly sit down and, in just under three weeks, try to draw up plans for bodies to reorder the world's finances in such a way as to obviate the causes of international conflict. As the next and subsequent chapters make clear, they were not entirely successful in this enterprise.

At that time the USA was by far the most powerful and undamaged nation in the world, and it was under the leadership of President Franklin Delano Roosevelt. He was a most remarkable man, passionate in his commitment to his country and to its people. To this day he is remembered by many people – not only Americans – with almost reverential affection. While many individuals and nations had been brought to the edge of economic ruin – and over it –during the Great Depression, he introduced the New Deal and such enterprises as the Tennessee Valley Authority. Thus his legislation brought financial salvation and security to millions of his own people. When he was 39 years of age, he was severely crippled with polio but, although he was wheelchair bound, this did not prevent him from becoming President in 1933 and from being re-elected three more times subsequently, in 1936, 1940 and 1944. He died of a brain haemorrhage in 1945.

His administration had consistently reflected his devotion to the ideal of the rights of ordinary people and his almost visceral detestation of royalty or anything that smacked of privilege gained by unearned wealth or social class. For that reason he felt an intense animosity towards the British Empire, which at the time constituted a serious check on US international trade and influence, by virtue of its complex matrix of tariff and trading arrangement with the British Empire. Hence on coming to office for the first time in 1933, Roosevelt made no secret of his desire to dismantle the British Empire and to aggressively promote US trading interests. Needless to say, many of the world's colonial people lauded the first of these aims, while more recently regretting his success in achieving the latter one!

It was in this context that Roosevelt, along with the famous English economist John Maynard Keynes (1883–1946), played such a pivotal role in setting up the two major economic bodies which today control the levers of global trade. These two bodies are the World Bank (officially called the International Bank for Reconstruction and Development) and the IMF. At Keynes' insistence, they were also about to set up a World Trade Organization (WTO) to ensure equity in international trade, as we shall see in Chapter 3, but Roosevelt eventually vetoed this idea because it would have imposed restraints on US economic power. As will also be explained in more detail in the next chapter, the WTO was eventually set up in 1995, but in such a way as to embrace US control over global trade, rather than the reverse.[16]

Roles of the World Bank and the IMF

The relationship between these two bodies is of immense importance to a consideration of what follows. It is summarised briefly below.

The IMF agrees on broad lines of policy in matters such as establishing and maintaining currency convertibility, and trying to avoid competitive exchange depreciation. In this sense, and unlike the World Bank, its main role was to be as a fiscal policy think tank and not merely a financial institution. Initially its basic financial policy was to adhere strictly to the gold standard in adjudicating loans to member countries. However, the USA came off the gold standard in the early 1960s, and thus the IMF was restrained from high-risk lending. Indeed, it only lends to treasuries and central banks of member countries, and generally over only five years. Originally, then, the IMF saw its function as to help member states in the short term should they run into temporary balance-of-payment problems.[17]

As we shall see in Chapter 3, it is the issue of which countries were 'member states' at Bretton Woods, and which ones are now, that has brought about a sea change. That is, the World Bank and the IMF were never intended to lend money to desperately poor 'peasant economies' of perennially low industrial capacity, but rather to nations – such as those in Europe – whose infrastructure had only been destroyed by the war.

Before discussing how the IMF could moderate short-term loans to temporarily cash-strapped nations, let us consider the IMF's twin sister, the World Bank. The World Bank has virtually the same membership as the IMF, but is endowed with much greater financial flexibility. For instance, it can make long-term loans over periods like 20 years, and can now even lend to private projects in less developed countries. As we shall see, it can – and frequently does – finance such private projects as setting up water purification facilities, in turn making it necessary for users to pay in order to access safe drinking water. In such ways, it is seen as directly influencing the running of poorer countries. The World Bank makes very wide use of private banks in both the developed and less developed world as principal and intermediary lenders. What is more, it can even sell outstanding debts on the financial markets. Indeed, it is this capacity of First World banks to 'sell outstanding debt' that keeps them safe, while mortgaging the LDCs even further.

The next chapter will explain more fully how the World Bank and the IMF became involved in lending money to very poor LDCs whose economies had never been strong and had not been ruined suddenly through war. The scenario unfolded as follows. From 1944 through 1972–73, the World Bank and the IMF loaned very little money to impoverished LDCs, especially those with no domestic oil reserves. However, the Organization of Petroleum Exporting Countries (OPEC) began to put pressure on the oil-hungry heavily industrial nations in Europe and North America by raising the price of oil. This brought huge profits in US dollars to the OPEC countries, which then invested them in developed country banks. These banks would then have to pay heavy interest rates on the deposits. Linked with the World Bank and the IMF, they then had to find some way of reinvesting the deposits to extract a higher interest rate than they would have to give to the original depositors. In effect LDCs, especially those which had no access to domestic supplies of oil, saved the banks in the developed world. The World Bank and the IMF shifted their interest to the LDCs, offering to make them development loans without too great regard as to whether or not the loans could ever be paid back without jeopardising the recipient country.

In order for them to repay, they needed to industrialise rapidly. This required the importation of oil from OPEC countries at high costs, which drove them to default on loan repayments and to ask for extensions on existing loans at even higher interest rates. Of course, now the banks were awash with US dollars that had to be reinvested quickly, and they were only too glad to help out in this way. Over time, this has led one LDC after another into an unbelievably perilous financial situation. For instance, some African countries are actually spending more on compound interest rates (not the principal!) than they can spend on health and education in their own countries. And it is here that the issues arises as to how the World Bank and the IMF can ensure that debt repayment is possible.

As soon as a loan is made by the IMF, the debtor nation has to agree to the structural adjustment policies (SAPs). These are conditions imposed by the banks on the country to ensure that its economy can maintain the repayments. Thus a common SAP requirement is that the debtor nation drastically reduces expenditure for government services. In any government, two major such services are health and education. Thus the debtor nation is compelled to privatise such services as far as possible. This leads to a great reduction in these services in the debtor country. Teachers and healthcare workers who were once employed in the public sector are dismissed and driven to seek employment in newly established private enterprise, which of course has to make a profit (which a public service is not required to do), and all of this causes a decline in working conditions in health and education as well as excluding a large proportion of the population from these services.

This is routinely coupled with what is referred to as 'verticalisation', which refers to the tendency to concentrate medical and educational services in the main urban/industrial areas, near ports, to further sustain the growing need of the debtor country to export goods for foreign sale in US dollars. All World Bank and IMF loans have to be paid off in US dollars. A country that is free to spend its resources on running health and education as public services will try to 'horizontalise' these services, the obvious aim being to reach all of its citizens. Thus increasingly after 1973, the IMF and the World Bank became accused of widening the gap in human rights between the developed countries and the less developed countries.

Role of the WTO

In closing this chapter, the author will now explain how the World Trade Organization (WTO) ties in with the World Bank and the IMF, and how its own mechanism to ensure compliance ties in with SAPs. As we have already seen, the type of WTO advocated by Keynes at Bretton Woods was rejected by the US President Roosevelt as an impediment to America's need to provide a global outreach for its huge and growing domestic industrial capacity, unchanged until then by the ravages of war or armed invasion. However, the WTO was reinstated in 1995, under terms more in harmony with the USA and in an attempt to give GATT more powers of re-enforcement.

Much more detail about the WTO and its impact on global health will be given in Chapter 3. For now it is only necessary to know that each country is theoretically represented in the WTO, and that the latter mediates trade regulations between countries, with the emphasis being on unfettered free trade. In pursuit of this it encourages various bilateral and multilateral agreements between countries to open up access to one another's markets – for instance, the North America Free Trade Agreement (which encourages Canada, the USA and Mexico not to tariff one another's industrial output), and the CARIFTA (the Caribbean Free Trade Association), which applies similarly to the small Caribbean countries, etc. However, two unilateral agreements that have been mediated and enforced by the WTO will be mentioned here as being of particular significance. They are the General Agreement on Tariffs and Trade (GATT) and the General Agreement on Trade in Services (GATS). GATT essentially gives the WTO the entitlement to insist on any country's right to export its goods to any other country. No country in the WTO has the right to try to protect its own products by imposing tariffs on imports. Even more draconian in its impact on health inequities between nations is GATS, which gives any WTO member the right to compete in selling services (such as health and education) to any other member state.

Both GATT and GATS have attracted a great deal of adverse comment over the last few years with regard to their negative impact on health, but any account of the WTO's arsenal in enforcing free trade would be incomplete if it did not mention Trade-Related Intellectual Property Rights (TRIPS). TRIPS is really a radical reinterpretation of patent law. It means that if a region is known to have traditionally been particularly successful in producing a particular crop, and if agronomists over time succeeded in isolating the particular gene complex and, better still, in reproducing it, they can patent it. Even if the original local producer wants to continue exporting its unique product, it can be charged a fee to do so under TRIPS regulations. This applies with equal force to naturally produced pharmaceuticals that local people may have been using for centuries. It certainly applies to pharmaceuticals isolated after years of research by large multinational houses. A telling example that has recently made the news is the production of antiretroviral drugs (ARVs) for the control of HIV/AIDS. Such pharmaceuticals are extremely expensive and cannot be routinely purchased by the vast majority of victims of HIV/AIDS in the less developed countries. However, both India and Brazil have recently earned a reputation for being able to mass produce generic copies of these expensive ARVs at as little as 4–5% of the normal cost. Yet TRIPS regulations under the WTO may well prevent the widespread sale of these generic copies to countries in Africa or elsewhere. This issue will be dealt with in detail in subsequent chapters.

One of the major criticisms of the WTO is that despite its democratic pretensions, its successive meetings have failed to address the needs of the less developed countries, objections to the adverse impact on health and other human rights of its rulings with respect to trade, and the application of TRIPS to medicine, agriculture, etc. To set the scene for further analysis of these pivotal issues, let us summarise the state of play.

A quick history of WTO resolutions

The purpose of the WTO, as already stated, is to bring about global free trade, and to this end the International Technical Barriers to Trade (TBT Agreement) was negotiated at the Uruguay round of GATT and then culminated in the Marrakech Agreement, out of which the creation of the WTO was actually negotiated in 1994. It formally came into existence on 1 January 1995. At the very first of its ministerial conferences (in Singapore in 1996), disagreements arose over the issues discussed previously between the delegates from the developed and less developed countries. They were not satisfactorily resolved, and were deferred for resolution at the Second Ministerial Conference (in Geneva in 1998). The debate was acrimonious, and it was decided to defer the issue until a new Director General had been elected. On 1 September 1999, Mike Moore (from the USA) assumed the post, but not without protracted argument. Another contender was Supachai Panithpakdi (from India), and a compromise was reached with the two sharing the post for three years each, Mike Moore holding the post first. Again, attempts to settle the concerns of the LDC delegates were deferred until the Third Ministerial Conference at Seattle in December 1999. It was during these deliberations that the now famous riots occurred, as popular antagonism to the WTO began to mount. The Seattle conference was followed in November 2001 by the Fourth Ministerial Conference in Doha, Qatar. At this conference the Doha Declaration was drawn up. This is a pivotal document that contains clauses purportedly designed to protect less developed nations from detrimental effects on health and trade arising from WTO rulings relating to TRIPS, etc. These clauses did not themselves have the force of law, and were sufficiently general in their formulation to make their enforcement ambiguous. For a more complete discussion of the Doha Declaration, the reader is referred to an earlier book by this author.[17]

Since the Doha Declaration, the WTO has been at the forefront of concern among people working for global equity in human rights, and its subsequent ministerial conferences have been anticipated with a mixture of cynicism that nothing will change and the hope that protective clauses will become binding. The Fifth Ministerial Conference took place in Taiwan in January 2002. However, the Doha Declaration barely got a look-in there, as the debate focused on the issue of customs and trading rights vis-à-vis China and Taiwan. China had finally become a member of the WTO a year earlier, in January 2001. The conference was on this occasion under the chairmanship of Supachai Panithpakdi, with the result that there was an expectation that perhaps the concerns of the LDCs would be given greater priority. Instead it was resolved that they would be discussed at the Sixth Ministerial Conference, to take place in Cancún, Mexico in September 2003!

At that meeting, an alliance of 22 delegates representing LDCs led by India, China and Brazil resisted developed world trading interests. In particular, they called for an end to agricultural subsidies within the EU and the USA. However, these talks also broke down, although there was agreement to solidify the Doha Declaration clauses at the next meeting. These delays of course continued to exacerbate the problems in the LDCs and, as we shall see, the health right inequities between the developed and less developed nations widened. Progress seemed to be made at the seventh ministerial conference in Geneva in August 2004. In summary, the agreement was that the EU and the USA, along with other developed countries, would lower agricultural subsidies. In exchange, the LDCs would lower tariff barriers to manufactured goods from the developed world.

To the casual reader, the significance of these concerns may seem remote from health rights issues. However, that is far from being so. Consider the case of Burkina Faso, one of the poorest nations in the world and a former French colony in Africa that achieved independence in 1960. Its soil and climate are such that it can produce prodigious crops of cotton cheaply and easily, and this is its principal export. However, in the USA, cotton farmers in Mississippi receive agricultural subsidies that allow them to use expensive fertilisers to produce cotton, not as easily as Burkina Faso does, but because of the subsidies the USA is able to sell what it does produce at an even lower price than Burkina Faso can on the international market. As Burkina Faso's cotton farmers face economic ruin, a precipitous derogation of domestic health and other human rights there is an obvious consequence.

So with regard to the Geneva Ministerial Conference, what has been the result? As we shall see in Chapter 3, the prevailing view is that it has been another thumbs down for the LDCs and their people. The well-known NGO, Oxfam, has condemned the Geneva meeting and the Eighth Ministerial Convention at Hong Kong in December 2005 as failing utterly to make meaningful decisions with regard to the Doha Declaration. Indeed, on 27 April 2006, that body called New Zealand (where it was meeting at the time) to do its bit with regard to reining in agricultural subsidies to help revive the Doha Development Goals.[18] Oxfam went on to say that the chances of a trade deal being done in 2006 that would help to reduce poverty were looking increasingly slim.

Oxfam's report, *A Recipe for Disaster*,[19] says that although a new deal is badly needed, the current offers are not good enough and poor countries would be better off missing the 2006 deadline and holding out for better offers. This is despite the fact that once the US administration loses its authority to negotiate trade deals without the involvement of Congress, a new deal could take years to agree.

References

1 United Nations. *From Concept to Convention: how human rights law evolves. Part 1, p. 1;* www.1.umn.edu/humanrts/edumat/hredustries/hereandnow (accessed 6 May 2006).

2 World Health Organization. *About WHO.* Geneva: World Health Organization; 2006; www.who.int/about.P.1 (accessed 6 May 2006).

3 MacDonald T. *Rethinking Health Promotion: a global approach.* London: Routledge; 1998.

4 Global Policy Forum, Peace Action International Office. *Convention on the Rights of the Child, Article 6 (Para 2) and Article 24 (Par 1);* www.globalpolicy.org/security/sanction/lawstds.httu (accessed 6 May 2006).

5 World Health Organization. *The Global Meeting on Future Strategic Directions for Primary Health Care: a framework for future strategic directions (Global Report – Alma Ata Declaration);* www.who.int/primary-health-care (accessed 6 May 2006).

6 Sanders D. *Primary health care and health system development: strategies for regeneration.* Paper presented at the International People's Health University, Cuenca, Ecuador, 11 July–24 July, 2005.

7 MacDonald T. *Health, Trade and Human Rights.* Oxford: Radcliffe Publishing; 2005. p. 3.

8 Seedhouse D. *Health Promotion: philosophy, prejudice and practice.* New York: John Wiley & Sons; 1997. p. 36.

9 Lalonde M. *A New Perspective on the Health of Canadians.* Ottawa: Information Canada; 1974.

10 United Nations. *Dr. Gro Harlem Brundtland.* UN press release, 29 June 1999; www.whop.org/inf-dg/biographies/gh-brundthland.html (accessed 6 May 2006).

11 Ibid., p. 11.

12 Brundtland GH. *Address to the Permanent Mission of the UN in Geneva*, 10 November 1998; www.people.brandeis.edu/~dwilliams/profiles/bruntland.htton (accessed 6 May 2006).

13 Bosely S. *Lee Jong-Wook – WHO Director.* Obituaries, *The Guardian,* 26 May 2006, p. 41.

14 World Health Organization. *3 By 5 HIV/AIDS Initiative.* Geneva: World Health Organization; 2005; www.who.int/hiv (accessed 6 May 2006).

15 Ibid., p. 15.

16 Rachman J, Bloch E, editors. *Multinational Corporations.* Chicago: Trade and the Dollar Publishers; 1974.

17 MacDonald T, op. cit., p. 15.

18 Oxfam. *Rich Country Greed Diminishes Prospect of WTO Deadline;* www.scoop.co.nz.stories/P0000604/500211.htm (accessed 6 May 2006).

19 www.oxfam.org.nz (accessed 6 May 2006).

Chapter 3

The global impact on human rights of UN agencies

The socio-political context of Bretton Woods

In order to understand how the various 'players' outlined in Chapter 2 on globalisation have impacted on health and human rights over time, and continue to do so, we will begin by taking a closer look at those fateful decisions taken at Bretton Woods in 1944. For one thing, it is important to realise that the less developed countries (LDCs) were largely unrepresented. Not only were virtually all of the countries represented major developed nations, but their agenda effectively meant that the reorganisation of the entire world economy would be necessary. The establishment of the World Bank and the IMF and, with them, the General Agreement on Tariffs and Trade (GATT), was the first time in human history that transnational institutions had been created specifically to solve practical global financial problems.

Not only did the horror and devastation of the Second World War itself impose a sense of urgency on the project, but overwhelmingly the opinion among the delegates was that pre-war problems had to be resolved in order to bring about an administratively feasible procedure for exercising transnational control over future events. Specifically, it was the majority view at that meeting that the emergence of fascism, especially in Italy, Spain and above all Germany, had been caused by the collapse of international trade and the tendency, especially in the USA, to indulge in isolationist economic policies. The Great Depression itself was held to have originated from the same causes as the rise of fascism.[1]

As has been described in Chapter 2, the US delegation played an extremely dominant role in the discussions and in determining the agenda for debate. In that sense, the presence of John Maynard Keynes from the UK proved to be somewhat of an irritant to the negotiations. He wanted to establish a world reserve currency administered by a central bank, itself to be set up by the Bretton Woods delegates. His argument was that this would create a more stable and certainly more impartial global economy by automatically recycling trade surplus in order to compensate for trade deficits. Such an idea was anathema to the interests of the USA. They wanted to run and referee global trade alone, and insisted that the only recognised tender be the US dollar, not some 'artificial world reserve currency' produced by a transnational central bank. However, before dealing with this issue, it is imperative to remember just how robust the US economy had become during the isolationist pre-war years. The wealth and welfare of citizens were tied to its huge industrial capacity and its flexibility and inventiveness in adapting to new industrial needs. Without unhindered global access to trade, its economy would be stifled.

Just to give an idea of how thrusting and vibrant that economy was, we are talking about a country that, towards the end of the Second World War, was turning out one fully equipped battleship a day![2] US fears back then were perfectly in keeping with the strongly isolationist tendencies that grew and fed into domestic politics between the world wars. It is important, in the author's view, to appreciate this because it renders current US resistance to such initiatives as an International Court of Justice and the Kyoto Environmental Global Protocols much more understandable. The latter are not instances of some newly hostile trend in US politics, but are deeply rooted in the country's cultural consciousness. Instead, the Conference made the fateful decision to impose a system based on both the freedom of movement of goods between countries and the use of the US dollar as the international currency. As we shall see, both of these policies underlie the global inequities with regard to health and human rights which so urgently need to be addressed. From those decisions arose the agreement that the IMF and the World Bank should be restricted to managing problems related to currency and capital shortage.

Original mandate of the IMF and the World Bank

It should now be obvious that the foregoing discussions were based on the assumption that the primary purpose of the IMF and the World Bank was to finance the restructuring of the war-wrecked economies of Europe. The idea of their role being to provide basic financial aid to the LDCs was not even considered. Indeed, as indicated in Chapter 2, the role of the LDCs as debtors to the two Bretton Woods institutions only came about through factors outside the control of that Conference.

The lack of a transnational central bank as suggested by Keynes meant that the IMF and the World Bank were not really 'banks' themselves with money to lend. They worked (and still do) through existing commercial banks largely in the USA and the UK. The application for a loan would be considered and handed over to one of the private banks involved for their discussion. The discussion was usually positive because, unlike personal loans, in which the bank manager has to decide whether the putative borrower is a good risk, a debtor country is almost always useful to have on your books. There are two main reasons for this. In the first place, the loan is made to the country, not to its leader. Thus if a country is run by a corrupt leadership that squanders the money on arms to keep its own populace down, or even fiddles and squirrels it away in Swiss bank accounts, and the government is then overthrown, the debt is still owed. The new regime, even if it is impeccably honest, is still liable. Secondly, and more to the point, in both the USA and the UK, if a debtor nation defaults, the bank's loss is made up by the Government. This is part of the arrangement that the IMF and the World Bank have with the participating private banks.[3] Not unnaturally, bank stockholders are rather partial to lending money to poor LDCs under these circumstances.

Private banks profit for the IMF and World Bank

In addition, the repayment programme to which the debtor nation agrees, and the attendant structural adjustment policies (SAPs), generate even greater profits for the lending bank. The repayments must be made in US dollars. To get these, the debtor nations generally have to export goods to wealthy developed countries. As part of the SAPs, the debtor nation has to buy from the lender nation any infrastructural equipment and/or services needed to industrialise production of the goods marketed. This, of course, does not only include the goods themselves, but the roads required to move the produce to the ports, the fertilisers required to increase yields, etc. Large-scale deforestation is often one of the attendant results. In addition, water supplies become chemically polluted, labour conditions deteriorate and union activity is suppressed in order to produce the export goods more cheaply. Typically, an LDC that is intensively producing a particular crop in order to finance repayments on its loan finds itself in cut-throat competition with other similar poor countries producing the same crop.

When such a debtor nation is unable to maintain payment of the compound interest[4] on the loan, it is usual for the loan to be rescheduled, which generates even more profit for the developed world lender nation's bank stockholders. As a result of these arrangements, the total international debt of the LDCs to the developed world has ballooned enormously. Fidel Castro, in one of his speeches, famously commented that 'La deuda internaccional es una deuda impagable' ('The international debt is an unpayable debt').[5] Further information about these matters can be found in the author's book, *Third World Health: hostage to First World wealth.*[6]

Entry into Europe of the Marshall Plan

Of course, as was indicated in Chapter 2, these problems did not become nearly so prominent until the 1970s, when the involvement of the IMF and the World Bank with the LDCs was reaching its height. And even in the comparatively halcyon days of 1945 to 1972, when the concern of these institutions was primarily with providing capital to put the war-ravaged European countries back on the track of economic recovery, those more experienced debtor nations began to resist. They especially disliked the way in which SAPs actually interfered with national policies on health, education and human rights. Because of this, the Marshall Plan was initiated. This plan was named after the American soldier and statesman, General George Marshall, who first proposed and strongly promoted the idea. Its aim was to provide US finance for European reconstruction mainly through grants rather than loans.

As implied above, of course, the poorer countries were not in a position to escape the harsh dictates of the SAPs, nor the degree to which those conditions were forcing them to mortgage the health and development of their own people. Especially compromised in this respect have been women and children, as will be described in subsequent chapters. Not only do such SAP policies as 'verticalisation' and the privatisation of health and education undermine the basic human rights of millions and widen the global equity gap, but also they have an adverse impact on trading power.[6] This comes about through the rulings of the WTO. WTO rulings also impact on nations in the developed world, but rarely as dramatically. A somewhat more trenchant perspective on the Marshall Plan can be found in Chapter 4.

The WTO and the tyranny of free trade

Greatly adding to the IMF-induced woes of LDC borrowers is the power of the WTO in enforcing free trade. Although all nations can be admitted as members to the WTO, all on a theoretically equal basis, this 'equality' is questionable. It is true that each WTO member has one seat, but there is no limit to the number of legal advisers that any nation can call upon in making its case to the WTO Council. This point is crucial, because most LDCs can only provide one 'adviser' (someone with specialist training in international law), while some have no such representation. The wealthier nations, on the other hand, may have several advisers, while the USA can provide dozens. The predictable effect is that, in a dispute between a small LDC and the USA over a free-trade issue, the USA is in a far stronger position to prevail.

However, despite this disadvantage, there are powerful voices in the developed world that seek to disempower LDC members of the WTO even further. Before considering this issue, it is important to realise that these poor nations were not entirely supine in their predicament.

The emergence of UNCTAD

The LDCs had begun to organise themselves and to demand better conditions by the early 1960s, when in Vietnam things were beginning to go badly for the interests of the USA. They could no longer so easily take the LDCs for granted. The cold war meant that the then USSR and the USA each worked assiduously to curry favour with the less developed nations. In this context, by 1965 the non-aligned nations had formed the Group of 77 to promote their grievances in UN circles. As a result, the UN Conference on Trade and Development (UNCTAD) was convened, and there the aggrieved LDCs were able to argue for more equitable terms for financing urgent development needs. The major developed nations could do little other than agree, but insisted that the Bretton Woods institutions would have to challenge any initiative arising from UNCTAD.[7] Of course the major developed nations, and particularly the USA, controlled the Bretton Woods institutions!

However, by 1968, the belief that the Bretton Woods committee could realistically run a global and stable monetary system based on fixed interest rates, with the US dollar as the only permitted international currency, was beginning to appear less and less plausible. Not only was this idea being resisted by both France and Germany, but also the US dollar was collapsing under the strain of war and budgeting deficits. Some of the smaller economies, such as Japan, were in vigorous ascendancy, and some LDCs had their self-confidence buoyed up by comparatively high growth rates and the above-mentioned dramatic increase in the price of oil. However, even that did not alter the balance of equity to the degree that was hoped and expected. Nations of the developed world responded by making many noble declarations of good intent at international forums both within and outside the UN, but without actually committing themselves to drastic change.

We have, of course, seen this many times since then, with successive G7/G8 resolutions to address the inequities and the dilatory tactics of the WTO in implementing the Doha Declaration being cases in point. We have already referred in passing to the enormous increase in dollar reserves accumulated in 1973 by the OPEC nations, and their tactic of investing these in the USA or the EU, according to a keynote editorial in the *New Internationalist* magazine.[1]

The enormous oil profits made by the OPEC nations in the 1970s (over US$ 310 billion from 1972 to 1977 alone) meant that the money had to be reinvested.

Most of it was deposited in commercial banks which, through the IMF, lent it to the non-oil-producing LDCs. The latter badly needed it to finance their major infrastructure projects that were being carried out for development. This increased the debt fivefold between 1973 and 1982. The amount owed reached US$ 612 billion, plus the high interest rates on the loans. Corruption saw to it that much of this money was filched by government personnel, and a great deal of it was spent on poorly planned projects. Countries like Mexico and Peru found themselves unable even to pay the mounting compound interest bills. Banks that were already in the IMF and the World Bank sold their outstanding debts to those bodies, which then imposed SAPs on the LDCs concerned, effectively taking over their economic policies.[8]

It is now undeniable that the World Bank and the IMF did take advantage of the situation at the time. Indeed, this was also consistent with the prevailing right-wing political context in the developed world, characterised by the policies of US President Ronald Reagan and UK Prime Minister Margaret Thatcher. All of these factors sustained what became the dominant orthodoxies of both the World Bank and the IMF, out of which grew the ideas of 'structural adjustment' and the various contradictions already discussed.

By 'structurally adjusting' the economies of the LDCs, they in effect deflated them because the SAPs required the borrower nation's government to use private services and to concentrate on production for dollar-earning exports, rather than for domestic consumption. This policy was highly profitable for the private banks, netting them US$ 178 billion between 1984 and 1990, but of course the LDC debt increased rapidly, and by 1992 it had reached US$ 1,300 billion, most of which was shifted to the IMF and the World Bank.

These policies allowed firms to take over the provision of such infrastructures in one LDC after another, such as the telephone and telecommunications services, and even the water supply, for which the country concerned then paid back in US dollars as part of the SAPs on which the loan was conditional. Delays in implementing the reforms promised at G8 and WTO meetings only highlight the problems. What this means, in effect, is that the IMF and the World Bank were taking more money out of the LDCs than they were putting back in! People in the LDCs, aware of this, often resisted their government's allying with the IMF by holding street riots, etc. Meanwhile, plans for World Bank-funded megastructures, such as dams, also encountered popular resistance due to the fact that citizens faced eviction from their homes and loss of their livelihoods. This has caused not only antipathy to western values, but also a parallel rise in religious fundamentalism and political violence.

In order to illustrate how this works in greater detail, Chapter 4 will deal with the issue and implications of privatisation of water supplies. However, before considering that, it is important to examine further the issue of the total impact of the Bretton Woods institutions on human rights as a whole. It is becoming increasingly clear that developed nations' financial power over the LDCs is by no means diminishing. Even the UN itself is becoming increasingly dominated by it. One has only to consider both the concentrated hostility to the UN, generated particularly in 2005, by the international media (controlled by the major developed countries' corporate wealth that runs the banks and the multinational firms that benefit from unfettered free trade), and at the same time the degree to which the UN is prevented from intervening effectively in situations involving gross violation of human rights.

The degree to which the UN is becoming deflected from its original human rights aims has been exemplified by a number of recent US moves. In August 2005, President Bush nominated John Bolten as US Ambassador to the UN. There was such strong opposition to the appointment within the USA that President Bush pushed through the nomination during the summer recess. The reason for this opposition by many thoughtful Americans was that they were aware of Bolten's barely disguised animus against the UN and his opposition to Kofi Annan. For these reasons, the appointment was regarded with apprehension by global health watchers throughout the world.

Bolten did not wait long (three weeks, in fact) to show his true colours. The 60th Annual Report of the UN was due in October 2005, and it had been intended that the Report would demonstrate that the gap in health, wealth and human rights between the LDCs and developed countries had widened significantly over the previous decade. It argued that this increase in poverty posed a growing threat to stability. On 26 August 2005, the Under-Secretary General for the UN Department of Economics and Social Affairs, Jose Antonio Ocampo, stated that the 2005 Report would focus on the international aspects of inequity, a decision reached by 191 member nations of the UN more than two years ago and on which over 100 of those countries have been actively involved in gathering data. It sounds alarm over the deepening disparities in health, education and economic participation between the developed world and the LDCs.

According to a UN press release dated 25 August 2005:

> Increasing poverty and the growing schism between the haves and have-nots will breed violence and terror if not reversed. This must include addressing economic asymmetries both within and between countries.

At present, 80% of the world's domestic product belongs to the 1 billion people in the wealthy countries, while the remaining 20% is shared by the 5 billion people in the LDCs. This is, of course, largely a legacy of economic neoliberalism and the current methods of monitoring international trade. The press release went on to note that this Report comes 10 years after the 1995 Copenhagen World Summit for Social Development, at which governments (including those of the UK and the USA) pledged to confront social challenges and to place people at the centre of development proposals. Focusing exclusively on economic growth as a developmental strategy appears to be ineffective.

John Bolten's response to this report has been to demand that it be largely scrapped. In other words, he is saying that the judgement of 191 other nations, elaborated over years of hard work, must give way to one nation's views after three weeks of analysis! His comments were summarised in a front-page article by David Usborne in *The Independent* of 26 August 2005. Usborne states that John Bolten wants to scupper the UN's global strategy with 750 amendments, even though the Report had been approved by Kofi Annan. In particular, the USA would delete any reference to the UN millennium goals on poverty, disease and inequity. Bolten also wants to eliminate the provision calling on nuclear powers to speed up disarmament, to remove agreed targets on foreign aid to the LDCs, to eliminate provisions to halt global warming, and to delete any references at all to the International Criminal Court, the world's only war crimes court. It is most interesting, in view of what we have already discussed with regard to the WTO and its powers, that he wants to restrict the joining of the WTO by LDCs! By way of additions, he wishes to highlight and amplify passages dealing with terrorism and the spread of democracy. Usborne ends his report with the rhetorical question: 'With Bush's man installed as US Ambassador to the UN, is this the end of diplomacy?'[9]

We shall return to a further consideration of an appropriate role for the UN in subsequent chapters, but first let us analyse in more detail the background to the slow and painful backdown in Hong Kong and elsewhere over the Doha Declaration.

Analysis of the Doha backdown

As of January 2007, it is becoming increasingly clear that the WTO Ministerial Conference has not satisfactorily resolved the issues raised in the Doha Declaration. The EU stiffened its opposition to possible restrictions on its agricultural policies by pushing, along with the USA, for even more conditionalities on LCD borrowings to become more open to imports of both goods and services from the developed countries. The Institute of Agriculture and Trade Policy (IATP) raised questions about food supply and the livelihood of agricultural workers in the LDCs, only to conclude that WTO policies will impact adversely on both of these concerns. In addition, the UNCTAD Mid-Term Reviews collapsed because of demands from the USA that it drop the issue of trade policy development from its mandate.[10]

Even more seriously, it is now clear that WTO policies actually undermine human rights. This claim is examined in detail in this chapter, where the point is put forward that even the way in which the WTO was established was in violation of the UN Charter on Human Rights. For now, though, let us consider how, by promoting trade liberalisation, the WTO has overridden efforts to improve the livelihood of the LDCs. This claim is made not only by the IATP, but also by the Third World Network (TWN) in their statement dated 22 December 2005.

In fine, it can be asserted that the long-awaited Hong Kong Ministerial has, in fact, disadvantaged the poorer nations. Their representatives lost on every count. The LDCs acceded to demands for key market access in services and in non-agricultural goods, but they did not gain significantly in cotton, aid for trade or market access in the developed countries. These were the three main components of the proposed 'development package.' With regard to the elimination of agricultural export subsidies by 2013, this was not really a gain. This subsidy was grossly unfair from the outset, and contrary to fair trade. The year 2013 was as far in the future as possible. Even 2010 would have been a disgrace, although that date was accepted by the LDC members.

What the rich and powerful countries really wanted from Hong Kong was to find ways of opening up LDC markets to developed country goods and services – and they eventually got their way at the end of the five days. The large transnational corporations are now preparing their governments to start multilateral negotiations involving key services, such as health and education. These multilateral requests were submitted by the end of February 2006. As if that was not enough, the final hours of the final day of the conference saw the developed nations extract huge concessions on the issue of non-agricultural market access (NAMA). Their NAMA agreements, when implemented, will severely de-industrialise the LDCs, retarding their development grossly. The strategies used at the last minute, especially by the EU delegate, Peter Mandelson, deserve some scrutiny. Mandelson threatened the LDCs with complete withdrawal from further negotiations if they did not agree to the NAMA proposals, and the latter gave the LDCs the impression that they did have something to gain by continuing discussions.

They did this rather deviously – and aided by the Secretariat – by offering different clusters of LDCs a specific advantage if they agreed. Then each specific interest group among the LDCs was given the impression that they would gain by acquiescence. This persuasive pressure was helped by the fact that only a few hours of conference time remained, and that the leaders of the G20 (India, Brazil and China), regarded as allies by many of the poorer countries, urged them to agree. Venezuela and Cuba were not convinced, but they could not persuade a sufficient number of the other LDCs of the merits of their opposition to NAMA.

By far the most negative outcome for the LDCs was in the area of services. The final outcome in this area invoked GATS, allowing developed nations' corporations to compete untrammelled in offering services (such as health and education) to desperate LDCs. Of course, the LDCs had put forward alternative proposals relating to services on the third day of the conference. However, these were rejected and did not appear in the final Ministerial Declaration, whereas the EU's amendments did.

The crucial aspect of the NAMA agreement is that it embodies what is known as the 'Swiss Formula.' The latter reverses the principle of less than full reciprocity by reducing the tariff of developed countries more than that of LDCs. This requires LDCs to embrace a tariff-reduction formula that affects all products, so it effectively dooms struggling industries in the LDCs. To gain some insight into the real impacts of the Hong Kong Ministerial, let us consider the issue of cotton. The Declaration agrees to end export subsidies in 2006, but these constitute only a small proportion of the US$ 9 billion with which the USA annually subsidises its cotton producers, while domestic subsidies constitute about 85% of the total US cotton support. No concrete action was agreed to address this. The same applies in the EU, where domestic subsidies comprise almost all of the cotton subsidies.

The African ministers were particularly anxious to address the cotton issue, and had demanded a cut of 80% on domestic cotton subsidies by 2006. What did the Hong Kong Ministerial Declaration say about this? It only endorsed the objective that, 'as an outcome of the negotiation, trade-distorting domestic subsidies for cotton production should be reduced.' Such a nebulous proposal is hardly sufficient. In addition, the LDCs had requested quota-free access to developed countries, but the latter would not agree to this! Therefore the Declaration avoided any such commitment.

Even with regard to product trading, the Ministerial Declaration includes an escape clause, offering almost no real protection for the LDCs. It states that if a developed country is having difficulty in providing total access to its markets, it need only offer 97% of products such access. In this way, developed countries can protect their domestic production of clothing, rice, sugar, leather goods and fisheries products. However, it is precisely these products which are of export advantage to LDCs.

For instance, only 2% of Japan's domestic produce is sensitive to LDC imports of these goods, so they are well covered by the 3% exemption. Likewise, the USA

---

*The 'Swiss Formula' is a widely used method for trying to narrow the gap between high and low tariff regions. Economists refer to this as 'harmonisation'. The 'Swiss Formula' was proposed by Switzerland at the Tokyo Conference on Tariffs in 1979.

has been able to allow clothing to be imported from either Bangladesh or Columbia. It all boils down to the fact that the LDCs can only have unfettered access to the developed world markets for products that they cannot produce at a low enough price – or not at all!

But what about UNCTAD? Wasn't it supposed to protect the interests of the LDCs?

The role of UNCTAD

This body has certainly tried to act as both an advocate and a mediator in trade-related issues for the LDCs, as is evident from comments by the Third World Network.[11] It is obvious that 'liberalising' trade does not create a level playing field, and has definitely not stimulated growth in service development in poor countries. In 2006, UNCTAD produced a similar paper, entitled 'Trade in Services and Development Implications', which was distributed at the Geneva meeting of its Commission on Trade in Goods and Services in February 2006.

This paper highlighted concerns about the impact of GATS and GATT, but especially the former. These included the displacement of local providers in favour of offshore firms, particularly in health, education and cultural provision. Basing much of its analysis on the outcome of the Hong Kong Ministerial, UNCTAD's paper stressed that even GATS and GATT allow for more flexible arrangements than the WTO seemed ready to acknowledge. The following points were mentioned in this context.

1 Liberalisation disadvantages the less favoured segments of the population, especially in essential services such as health.
2 Trade liberalisation can undercut a nation's own, long evolved values in cultural and educational matters.
3 Trade liberalisation creates short-term costs, which distort national planning.
4 Some services, as currently provided domestically, need time to adjust to the international market before they can become competitive.

What UNCTAD suggests is that each country has unique needs and contexts with regard to commodity and service provision, and should be allowed time to access the costs and benefits involved before being forced to comply with GATS and GATT. This must involve such issues as employment displacement vs. employment creation, provision for technology instruction, gains in efficiency vs. negative impacts on the informal sector, raising quality standards to allow effective competition in overseas markets, etc. Barriers posed by international standards, development of infrastructures and means of facilitating market access, etc., also need time and scope for development.

The paper addresses a wide range of findings on a variety of sectors not directly related to health or other human rights, but they are most certainly indirectly related. For example, a study of Ecuador, which has been badly affected since 2005 by the 'dollarisation' of the economy to bring it into line with the requirements of bilateral trade agreement and of GATS, showed that in distribution of services it is crucial to avoid a market situation in which the product (or service) of several sellers is in the interests of one buyer! That problem arose in Ecuador's wholesale services. If liberalisation of trade took place under such conditions, it would merely replace a monopoly of domestic providers with a foreign monopoly.

Africa signals erosion of UNCTAD

As is so often the case, some of the African countries seem to suffer the most at the hands of global finance. And it is African trade ministers who have been most vocal in commenting on UNCTAD's apparent loss of influence. Moreover, they strongly argue that developed world interests are complicit in this. This issue was extensively debated in Nairobi in April 2006 at the fourth session of the African Union's Conference of Trade Ministers. Indeed, concern was so great that a special motion on UNCTAD, and possible reforms to it, was adopted by the conference.[12]

'We know that UNCTAD has come under pressure, and we need a vote of confidence on UNCTAD and to send it a signal of solidarity', the Kenyan Trade and Industry Minister, Mukhisa Kituyi, said. One of the Zimbabwean delegates was even less optimistic when he observed that reforms to the UN that were gathering pace in New York could even threaten the survival of UNCTAD.

Proposals voicing such concerns were supported by other delegations, including those from Zambia, Lesotho and Ghana. The ministers presented a Declaration which included the statement that:

> In view of the nature of UNCTAD's programmes and activities for capacity building, we are concerned with recent proposals of some developed countries to erode the mandate of UNCTAD or even to discontinue it altogether.[13]

Such warning signals arise in the context of a movement among corporate interests in some developed countries to radically restructure the UN so that its activities bring it more into line with neoliberal financial control. The Netherlands, Belgium and the UK, with US approval, are proposing that UNCTAD's influence be diluted by merging it with other agencies. One version of this, for instance, would see UNCTAD merged with the WTO or the UNDP, or even into a single UN Development Authority.

The hidden face of developed world financial power

What must be realised is that, catastrophic as the financial plight of the LDCs is, it fits in brilliantly with the needs of developed world business interests. Only six weeks prior to the 'Millennium Round' in Seattle, the US Senate had approved deregulation of the country's banking system! This would make it legal for US banks and transnational corporations to invest heavily in other countries. The implications are clear. A small cluster of US financial bodies will gain control over the entire US financial services industry. It should come as no surprise that these are the bodies that would benefit most from financial services deregulation under GATS. These enormously powerful financial bodies will end up overseeing financial and economic development globally. They are the creditors and shareholders of high-tech manufacturing, the defence industry, major oil and mining interests, etc.

Because they would underwrite public debt, they would have an effective control on individual politicians and even of governments. They could determine whether or not it is to their financial advantage to declare war, for instance, and because of the matrix of organisational connections, are in a position to mediate its prosecution.[14]

Furthermore, the clauses of the now defunct Multilateral Agreement of Investments (MAI), which was to provide 'national treatment to foreign banks', are in the process of becoming a fait accompli. They are fully integrated with insurance companies which themselves oversee multinational healthcare providers, such as those that the present UK government under Prime Minister Tony Blair is anxious to involve in the National Health Service of Britain. In the USA, these same providers are actively lobbying for the deregulation of public healthcare under GATS. This threatens the entire welfare state and could nullify most of the great social gains that have been achieved since 1945.

Possible impact on the UK's National Health Service

Since 1947, Britain has been blessed with its NHS – brought into being after the Second World War and honed over the years since then. It allows every UK citizen access to all levels of healthcare, most of it free at the point of contact. However, the present government, as part of its desire to become more integrated with US policies, has been making moves to gradually privatise the NHS and thus bring it under neoliberal financial deregulation. It is doing this in various ways, one of the most prominent being various Private Finance Initiative (PFI) schemes. Under the present NHS, whatever its inefficiencies, the entire UK population is covered and it costs less than 7% of the gross national product (GNP).

The US spends far more (nearly 15% of the GNP) under its system, which relies largely on health cover from private health insurance funds. There are also government-funded programmes that give financial aid to the elderly and disabled, but these are nowhere near complete, and in any case they do not cover all illnesses. On top of this, about 31% of Americans have no health insurance cover at all. Basically, UK citizens seem to get a lot more for their 7% of GNP than US citizens do for their 15%!

However, the NHS and organisations like it are anathema to neoliberal orthodoxies. The case has been well and succinctly argued by Dr Hannah Caller.[15] It turns out that the hospitals worst affected by bad management, ward closures, reductions in staff, etc., were those under the PFI. The Centre for International Public Health Policy at the University of Edinburgh has analysed the performance of eight of the PFI schemes. It showed that the proportion of their annual reserves devoted to servicing capital expenditure rose from 4.5% to 16% as a result of the introduction of the PFI.

Already a number of large multinational finance corporations are involved in the PFI, or are hungrily waiting by the sidelines, because there are large profits to be made from healthcare under GATS. However, it stands to reason that if profits are made by it (which they are), these dividends must come out of funds that would otherwise all pay for healthcare. It is difficult to see how people can credit any argument to the contrary, but certainly a great deal of money is being spent in order to try to persuade them. It is in the interest of corporate power that the PFI battle be won in the UK.

Corporate involvement in the UK's NHS is comparatively slight so far, but even so, juicy profits have already been made. Caller cites an example. Two years after completion of the Norfolk and Norwich PFI hospitals, four finance corporations – Barclays Bank, Stereo, Innisfree and John Laing – decided to refinance their joint working company, Octagon. This alone allowed them to make a profit of

£115 million (close to US$ 200 million). They gave £45 million to the hospital, and kept the rest! This increased their rate of return from 16% to 60%. The NHS health trust currently saddled with this arrangement would have to pay £257 million to extricate itself from it. Even now, in order to pay the PFI consortia, the hospitals concerned have had to reduce beds by 25% and staff by 15%.

Two points clearly emerge from the above discussion. First, neoliberal finance does not victimise only the LDCs. The UK is most certainly a highly developed society, but once it allows itself to become so closely tied to neoliberalism, its own citizens are spared no more than LDC citizens, nor are the US citizens spared. Secondly, if health is to be a basic human right, there is no room for financial profits to be made out of its provision. Financial deregulation in the USA threatens human rights globally.

First the USA and then the world

From what we have seen so far, financial deregulation in the USA is an inducement – the profit motive – to apply it anywhere. The Millennium Round in Seattle, by calling for deregulation of capital movements, gives greater legitimacy to speculative trade and hence tightens the grip of neoliberal financial control.

Control over the channels of speculative trade confers on financial corporations in the developed countries, especially the USA and countries in the EU, the power to manipulate currency and hence stock markets. It even impairs the role of central banks globally. Consider the 'Asian Crisis' of 1997. More than US$ 100 million were effectively confiscated from Asia's central banks. Russia and Brazil suffered similar assaults in 1998 and 1999, respectively. Moreover, the IMF played a key role in mediating these assaults.

Iraq and other wars: accident or consequence

In the light of the following, it is not difficult to see how wars fit in with the neoliberal global finance agenda. All we have to do is to ask what happens to countries that refuse to deregulate trade and foreign investment and to allow 'national treatment' to multinational corporations (MNCs) and banks of the developed world. The USA, and the developed world military intelligence, routinely interferes with financial affairs. The IMF, the World Bank and the WTO, which police economic reform globally, find no difficulty in cooperating with NATO and similar agencies in 'peace-keeping' endeavours. In the same way, the financing of post-conflict restoration easily fits in with that agenda, much to the profit of developed world stockholders.

As we enter the third millennium, war and the free market go hand in hand. War physically destroys whatever has not been dismantled through deregulation, and provides 'national treatment' to banks and corporations in the developed nations. Thus although the Seattle Round purportedly set out to 'peacefully' re-colonise many LDCs by manipulating market forces, it has not hesitated to call on military support as required. Therefore war and financial globalisation should not be seen as separate issues. This means that opposition to the WTO would be more effective if it was linked, in various countries, with the growing anti-war movement.

What all of this means, in effect, is that the WTO cannot be regarded as part of any plan to guarantee existing human rights – or as being engaged in the effort to extend them. As we have seen, under WTO rules, the banks and MNCs can legally distort LDCs' economies to the advantage of their First World stockholders. This really is a new and more efficient method of colonisation. Baldly speaking, the WTO rules legitimise the actions of global banks, MNCs, etc., in destabilising Third World institutions, bankrupting their producers and taking over the economies of small countries. In effect, they put into operation a triangular division of authority between the WTO, the IMF and the World Bank that can create a system of 'global surveillance' of developing countries, their economies and even their social policies.

The clear implication of this is that the policies of the IMF and the World Bank will reign without notice of any ad hoc country-level loan agreements. In fact, the rulings of the IMF will, in time, become permanently established under the Seattle Millennium Round. Such countries will, in effect, be permanently in debt to the most powerful business syndicates in the world. The WTO's role will then be to police the enforcement of the SAPs, and all according to international law!

Prospects for a new UN Human Rights Council

Certainly the evidence presented so far in this chapter indicates that although the IMF, the World Bank and the WTO are agencies of the UN, their combined impact does not appear to have been unambiguously supportive of the human rights components of the UN Charter. The intervention of the UN was in fact to readdress the entire issue of human rights by establishing a new Human Rights Council at a meeting during March 2006, to replace the existing Human Rights Commission. However, after many months of discussion, a solution appeared to be at hand, until US intervention – in the now familiar form of John Bolten – derailed the process. On 23 February 2006, Jan Eliasson, the UN General Assembly President, issued a preliminary version of the resolution for the assembly to adopt at its March meeting. At that point the US ambassador to the UN announced that the USA opposed the draft and preferred negotiations to continue.

It was not only LDC governments that had been supportive of the proposal, but also many developed world governments, including members of the EU. Thus the US opposition greatly annoyed the UN Secretary General, Kofi Annan. He had been strongly advocating acceptance of the resolution and was quoted as saying, 'I am chagrined about the US position and I urge the US to find some way of associating itself with the majority of the member states.'[16]

The initial move to change the Human Rights Commission had in fact been made by the EU in order to strengthen the UN's human rights work and to ensure that countries with a bad human rights record could not become members. The Commission has 53 members, and elections have been through regional groupings. In September 2005, the UN agreed 'in principle' that the Commission would be replaced by a new Human Rights Council. However, disagreements arose over the Council's mandate. In particular, there was heated argument as to how members of the new body would be elected. The choice was whether to do this by a simple majority or by two-thirds of the General Assembly. Other contentious issues included how many members would be allocated from each region, whether countries with poor records on human rights could be eligible, how periodic reviews of a country's human rights performance would be mediated, and so on, as well as whether NGOs should have a say on the human rights credentials of putative members. A compromise was finally reached, as incorporated in the General Assembly President's draft in February (as mentioned above), and it was generally assumed that it would be accepted, until John Bolten rejected it.

Bolten's major objection centred on the issue that countries with poor human rights records can still get a place on the Council. However, this objection is rather embarrassing because many Assembly Members regard the USA itself as having a poor human rights record, not least because of the questionable legitimacy of its treatment of inmates in its prison at Guantanamo Bay. The draft proposal envisions a geographical distribution of council members as follows: Africa, 13; Asia, 13; Eastern Europe, 6; Latin America and the Caribbean, 8; Western Europe and Other States Group, 7. As the reader will note, this procedure would fit in well with the author's suggestion, in the final chapter of this book, that such a regionally based council should mediate global regional trade protocol.

The General Assembly President, Jan Eliasson, indicated other key differences to the proposed Council over the Commission.[17]

- The Council would have a renewed focus on dialogue and cooperation.
- The Council would meet regularly throughout the year and have mechanisms for convening additional sessions if necessary.
- The Universal Periodic Review would allow for assessment of each state's fulfilment of its human rights obligations.
- Allocation of seats would be according to equitable geographical distribution.
- Members of the Council would not be eligible for immediate re-election after two consecutive terms.
- Although membership of the Council would be open to all UN Member States, there would be legitimate expectations on members, as the General Assembly can suspend a Council member that commits gross and systematic violation of human rights.

As outlined in the March 2006 draft, elections to the Council would have been held on 9 May 2006, and the first meeting of the Council would have been convened on 19 June 2006. Three days earlier, on 16 June 2006, it was proposed that the existing UN Commission on Human Rights should be abolished. However, the US objection has of course thrown the whole procedure into confusion. On 13 March 2006, the Commission on Human Rights met for its annual session, but the issue was not clarified there. This substantiates the growing view that there is nothing benign about the effects and intentions of the USA, or other powerful First World nations, and the huge transnational business interests that they represent, with regard to the mediation of global human rights. It is becoming increasingly clear that the bottom line is the financial interests of First World banks and corporations. If human rights anywhere come into conflict with these, then the banks and corporations dominate. In this author's view, this represents a clear violation of the original UN Charter.

References

1 Swift R. Squeezing the south: fifty years is enough. Keynote editorial. *New Internationalist*, July 1994 issue, pp. 4–7.
2 Hubeman L, Sweezy P. *Introduction to Socialism.* New York: Modern Reader; 1968. p. iii.

3 MacDonald T. *Third World Health: hostage to First World wealth.* Oxford: Radcliffe Publishing; 2005. p. 48.

4 Ibid., pp. 241–3.

5 MacDonald T. *A Developmental Analysis of Cuba's Health Care System 1959.* Lewiston, NY: Edwin Mellen Press; 1999. p. 22.

6 MacDonald T (2005), op. cit., p. 153.

7 United Nations. *Formation of UNCTAD.* Conference on Trade and Development; http://en.wikipedia.org/wiki/New International Economic Order (accessed 9 November 2006)

8 Ibid, p. 7.

9 Usborne D. The US vs. the UN. *The Independent,* 26 August 2005, p. 8.

10 Institute of Agriculture and Trade Policy. *Why is the Doha Round Failing?;* www.tradeobservatory.org/html (accessed 19 June 2006).

11 Khor M. UNCTAD raises development concerns on service liberalisation; www.twnside.org.sg/title2/twinfo348.htm (accessed 19 June 2006).

12 Third World Network. African Ministers warn against erosion of UNCTAD's mandate; www.twnside.org.sg/title2.twinfo391.htm (accessed 19 June 2006).

13 Chessudovsky M. WTO – an illegal organization that violates the Universal Declaration of Human Rights; www.derechos.org/nizkor/articlulos/chossudovskye.html (accessed 19 June 2006).

14 Ibid., p. 9.

15 Caller H. 'Health matters': fight racism – fight imperialism. *Organ of the Revolutionary Communist Group,* June/July issue 2006, p. 3.

16 Khor M. Birth pangs of UN's New Human Rights Council. Global trends; www.twnside.org.sg/gtrends.htm (accessed 19 June 2006).

17 Caller H, op. cit., p. 3.

Chapter 4

Worsening global equity of access to safe water

Safe water: crucial to health rights

Health depends on access to many things – food, shelter, water, and so on, and even positive self-esteem – but of all of these water is the most basic need. In 1920, during the Irish resistance to British rule, the Mayor of Cork, Terence MacSwiney, was arrested by the English. He died in Brixton Prison after a 74-day hunger strike, but *he was drinking water regularly*. Without water we know that he would have died far sooner. We must regard water as a fundamental component of the basic human right of health. Without it, the presence of the best and most ample of the other requirements referred to above would be useless.

However, let us be clear about one thing. The right of access to safe and potable water was not officially recognised as a 'basic human right' until November 2002.[1] This being so, there can be no question of it taking second place to financial considerations. The Office of the High Commission for Human Rights amended the International Covenant on Economics, Social and Cultural Rights (ICESCR) to include the right to water under Article 11 (the right to adequate standard of living) and Article 12 (the right to health) as a result of General Comment 15, and it was ratified by 145 countries. It states that:

> The human right to water entitles every person to sufficient, affordable, physically accessible, safe and acceptable water for personal and domestic uses.

The Covenant goes on to specify that all governments must embrace national strategies to bring this about.

The natural distribution of safe and potable water over the surface of the globe, and among its various peoples, is very unequal to begin with. With modern technology we can often 'make deserts bloom' and enable people to live in areas that were formerly hostile to life, but the application of this technology has been rather patchy, and on the whole the technology applied to water supplies has had the effect of making them less accessible to more people. Before we consider the inequitable access to water technology, let us look at the current situation with regard to large-scale deflection of water from the many for the recreation of the few.

Hotels, and their attached golf courses, are as good a place to start as any. Golf-course management requires extraordinary quantities of fresh water, and some lavish clubs established in poorer countries for the use of wealthy tourists threaten the health of local people in parts of the world as far apart as Fiji, North and South America, many African countries, Jamaica, the Philippines and large parts of Asia. Even in developed countries, such a profligate waste of water and of the maintenance of the necessary reticulation technology is now causing concern. Giles Trimlett, a *Guardian* newspaper reporter, has commented on the situation with regard to the serious abrogation of health rights in the Philippines.[2]

Such facilities are extremely costly to maintain at the local level, but are of little benefit to the people who pay for them. In this context I am not referring to the direct cash costs so much as the severe undermining of health and other human rights. When a large hotel with a golf course is built, this is often in an area in which thousands of people are living on land in a relatively 'unofficial' fashion and in dwellings that may not have been properly planned. Such people are often the poorest of the poor, who have migrated from rural areas in search of jobs. As soon as the land they live on has been designated as a tourist facility, their previously free supplies of water from pumps are cut off.

In the southern Mediterranean region there were about 200 golf courses in 2003, each of which would consume the same amount of fresh water as a town of 1,200 people, according to a World Wide Fund for Nature report in 2004. South-east Spain is already an arid region, but 89 more golf courses are planned as the tourist trade there booms. Likewise, Greece is planning 40 more and Cyprus 8 more golf courses. The report's author, Lucia de Stefano, describes the region as wilting under the pressure caused by 135 million tourists' use of beach-side resorts extending from northern Morocco and Spain to Greece and Turkey, Cyprus and Tunisia. She estimated that this figure would double by 2006.[3]

Water, water, everywhere – but not to drink

We are thus secure in asserting that fresh water is not a commodity to be taken for granted worldwide. Few people in the LDCs have it on tap, and many of those who do have no guarantee of its potability and freedom from infection. In most of the places in which the author has been privileged to be of service, all except the very wealthy have had to carry water for domestic necessities for long distances. Diarrhoea caused by infected water kills large numbers of infants and frail elderly people. These deaths – and the inconsolable suffering attendant on them – are largely preventable, but not under the present inbuilt inequities between the wealthy and the poor nations.

Even in countries such as the Dominican Republic, a major tourist spot for wealthy people, tap water is unsafe. The wealthy buy safe water in large bottles which are regularly delivered to hotels and to their homes, but the great majority of the population routinely experiences typhoid and other waterborne diseases. Death by such causes is so common, yet within hailing distance of thoughtless pleasure-seekers, who know nothing about it. The ostentatious displays of wealth in that country have to be seen to be believed. While working there in medicine between 1985 and 1987, I constantly met up with tourists and the local wealthy expatriate community who resolutely did not want to know what was happening so close at hand. They were 'enjoying themselves' and found such information 'unsettling.' They would return to the USA, the UK or elsewhere and enthuse about how lovely the Dominican Republic was. The degraded lives of the dispossessed had nothing to do with them. In a fair world, of course, such attitudes can have no place. Let us now take a brief historical look at the development of our relationship with the planet's water supply.

Growing developed world control over water

Before the European 'Industrial Revolution' of the eighteenth and nineteenth centuries, people everywhere had a somewhat similar association with water. They relied almost exclusively on water available at, or near, the surface of the earth. Rivers, lakes and springs constituted the most commonly used sources. Indeed, it was widely assumed that these sources were inexhaustible, due to the evaporation–rain cycle. However, in Europe and North America, rapid industrialisation quickly changed all that. Large quantities of the easily accessible water were needed to run generators and other machinery. River sources – and more recently ocean coastlines – became polluted and unfit for use. Sewerage systems became necessary as larger concentrations of people grew up around ports and factories. In the developed world, we began our long-term exploitation of underground water resources (aquifers, which are water-bearing rocks, or rock complexes, underground) and even the elaboration of huge desalination enterprises.

As Nares Craig[4] has pointed out, the developed countries and even some LDCs are now exploiting the aquifers at a prodigious rate. Without some kind of international mediation and control, it is difficult to see how this can continue. Aquifers contain about 97% of the planet's water supply. Increasingly these very sources face the risk of pollution. However, merely their rate of use must be cause for alarm. Water tables are now dropping at the rate of 3 metres annually, according to some estimates. In the prairie states of the USA and the prairie provinces of Canada, up to 15 metres of water are being extracted annually, while the natural replacement rate of 1 cm per year is only $^1/_{1500}$ of that!

It is anticipated that aquifer sources of water in North America and Australia will be exhausted by about 2013. Of course, the impact of all this will not be felt first or most adversely in the developed world, but in the nations of the less developed world. As Craig points out,[5] in Beijing province, and in two neighbouring provinces, over 100,000 aquifers had run dry by 2000. Worse still, the use on an industrial scale of this non-renewable resource strictly for profit in the developed world is increasing year by year. This has to be curbed, and soon. Even some people in the developed world are now imminently threatened by it, but of course it is the poor who bear the greatest brunt.

In this context it struck me as perversely ironic when in June 2006 I received an email advertisement for a private water supply firm on the lookout for aid agencies willing to promote its product. From the advertisement, I quote the following:

> As of 2006 it is estimated that one person in five has no access at all to safe drinking water and at least 5,000 children die every day from waterborne diseases. Moreover, it has been estimated that by 2020 we will need about 17% more water in total than will be available.[6]

As will become evident later in this chapter, using figures from more reliable academic and government sources, the data quoted in this advertisement may well understate the case! However, before we deal with these sources more analytically, it is important to be clear about the term 'safe' when applied by these agencies as an adjective to describe water. Water that is clearly fit for human consumption is referred to as 'potable' or drinkable, but the term 'safe' is much broader. Water that is not ordinarily intended for drinking, but which is not harmful if used in boiling food, is referred to as 'safe.'

On 2 December 2005, the United Nations Children's Fund released a report on the issue of global access to water. It pointed out the following alarming statistics. In mid-2006, nearly 40% of the world's people (almost 2.5 billion people) did not have regular access to sanitation facilities. Of these people, 300 million live in Africa. In the LDCs, most waste water (about 90%) is not treated before it is poured directly into rivers and streams used by people for drinking, bathing, etc. This gives an immense boost to waterborne diseases, many of which are lethal and to which children are especially vulnerable. In fact, in the LDCs, 80% of illnesses and deaths are attributed to such diseases, taking an average of one child's life every 8 seconds.[7]

If such water is used for bathing, it causes a host of unpleasant skin diseases. Eye infections, such as trachoma, are a particularly common phenomenon. Trachoma leads to an intensely painful scabbing of the cornea and is a major source of blindness. It is estimated that six million people (virtually all of whom live either in LDCs or in grossly underdeveloped parts of developed countries) suffer from trachoma. In Australia, many Aborigine communities contend with this disease – and all of its attendant consequences, such as lack of access to literacy. Women are twice as vulnerable to this distressing condition as men.

An NGO that has particularly distinguished itself with regard to collating information on the privatisation of water services and supply in the LDCs is the World Development Movement (WDM).[8] It produces regular reports on progress made – or not made – in urging governments to assume responsibility for ensuing universal access to safe water, rather than allowing it to become a privatised commodity and a victim of WTO GATS regulation. More will be said about this later in this chapter, but let us now consider the general issue of the extent to which there is access to safe and reliable sources of water across the globe in general. That is, what are the present politics of water?

Politics of water: a conspectus

Populations all over the world are expanding, and this, together with the consequent increases in pollution, etc., means that per-capita access to water is decreasing. This is increasingly making water a key element in a number of conflicts. Many observers have commented that a nation's possession of water will, in the future, be a strong determinant of its international standing. On that basis, Canada could become the world's richest country. However, not all of this is recent, and for many centuries wars have been fought either directly over water resources or as a result of disputes over access to ports, etc.

In 2003, the UNESCO World Water Development Report (WWDR) argued that in the next two decades water quality worldwide will decrease by 30%. It states that 40% of the world's people currently do not have sufficient water to meet the needs of basic hygiene.[7] In 2000, 2.2 million or more people died either from using contaminated water or as a result of drought. A UK-based NGO, Water Aid, reported in 2004 that one child dies every 15 seconds because of water-related diseases.

The USA easily leads the world in water consumption, which amounts to 2,000 cubic metres per person per year. Much of this is used up on golf courses, in car washing, etc. Canada comes second, at 1,600 cubic metres per person per year. The latter figure is about twice what the French use, three times what the Germans use, and almost eight times what the Danish use. Once we move from OECD nations to LDCs, the differences are much greater. Even worse, though, the Canadian figure represents an increase of almost 28% since 1980. The nine OECD countries, by contrast, have decreased their total water use since 1980.[9] These OECD nations are the Czech Republic, Denmark, Finland, Luxembourg, the Netherlands, Poland, Sweden, the UK and the USA.[10]

In the USA, about 9.5% of fresh water is underground. The largest such holding is the Ogallala Aquifer, which is 1,300 km long and extends from South Dakota to Texas. It irrigates 20% of US farmland. This aquifer was formed over a million years ago, but in the last century has been cut off from its original sources and is now being used up at the rate of 12 billion m³/year. Indeed, some experts predict that it will be exhausted by 2030.[10] Mexico City shares a water problem with London, England, in that about 40% of the city's water is lost through leaking pipes built in 1901.[11] London's leaks are also prodigious, some in piping that was laid in Victorian times.

Rich in oil, poor in water

The author has had the privilege of serving in Libya, and it is in the Middle East that one has the bizarre experience of living in one of the richest areas in the world, where virtually anything can be bought, yet where life hangs on a mere trickle of water. In fact, the region only has 1% of the world's freshwater supply, while being home to 5% or more of the world's population. Thus in this area of the world water is considered to be a strategic resource. It has been estimated that by 2025 the countries of the Arabian Peninsula will require more than twice the amount of water that is naturally available.[12] Two-thirds of the Arab nations have to get by on less than 1,000 m³ of water per person per year, and this is considered to be the limit.[13]

Consider the predicament of Jordan, which had little water to begin with, a situation that has been worsened by dam building. However, this country is also a victim of Israeli politics. The 1994 Israel–Jordan Peace Treaty involved Israel agreeing to give 50 million m³ of water per year to Jordan, but it refused to do so in 1999, and then withdrew from the Treaty. It was in keeping with that 1994 treaty that Jordan built the dams in the first place.[14] This lack of water has forced Jordan to develop techniques for reusing second-hand water and to set up desalination units. The latter are prodigiously expensive to operate. For instance, the Disi Groundwater Project in the south of Jordan will cost US$ 250 million.

Another proposed major project, which would help if they could get it going, is the Unity Dam on the Yarmouk River. This dam was started in 1987 and would benefit both Jordan and Syria, but the project could not be completed because it was opposed by Israel.[15] Although both Israel and Jordan need the Jordan River, it is controlled by Israel, along with 10% of the rest of the water in the region.

In addition, water plays a pivotal role in the conflict between Israel and the Palestinian Authority. Indeed, Israel's former Prime Minister, Ariel Sharon, was quoted on the BBC as saying that it was one of the causes of the Six Day War! Abel Darwish, on the same programme, also said, 'The Israeli army is in control over the water supply and prohibits Palestinians from pumping water while "settlers" do so, and use much more sophisticated pumping techniques than Palestinians can afford.' Palestinians, according to Darwish's report, complain that Israel uses about 80% of the underground water.[16] Israelis in the West Bank use four times as much water as their Palestinian cohabitants.[17] The World Bank estimates that 90% of the water in the West Bank is the West Bank's water. In this regard, it is interesting that Article 40 (Appendix B) of the Oslo Accords states that Israel recognises Palestinian rights to water in the West Bank.

The Golan region of Syria also provides Israel with 770 million m^3 of water per year – this represents one-third of its total consumption. The Golan water table goes to the Sea of Galilee, Israel's largest reserve. However, Golan has been occupied by Israel since 1967 and, because of the water alone, represents a strategic territory for Israel. The level of the Sea of Galilee has been falling fast and there is now real concern that Israel's main water reserve will become salinated. Then, on its northern border with Lebanon, Israel almost went to war in 2002 when Lebanon opened a new pumping station that took water from a river feeding the Jordan River. To avert the crisis, Israel began to investigate the possibility of building desalination plants.[18]

In the mean time, Turkey caused consternation in both Iraq and Syria when it started construction of the Ataturk Dam and an ancillary system of 22 dams on the Tigris and Euphrates rivers in 1990. BBC Radio asserted that the number of 'water-poor' countries in the region increased from three in 1955 to eight in 1990, with another seven expected by 2010.[19] All of this adds a new perspective of urgency to resolving the Middle East crisis as quickly as possible.

Let us briefly switch our attention to Asia, where China's huge Three-Gorges Dam is causing concern to both Vietnam and Cambodia. This will be one of the world's largest dams and a source of multiple environmental problems. In addition, China is anxious to divert water from the Yangtze River to the rapidly dwindling Yellow River because the latter is the principal source of irrigation for China's wheat-growing regions.

Further south, exploitation of the Ganges River is the subject of dispute between India and Bangladesh. Water reserves are dwindling and becoming polluted, while the glacier that feeds the Ganges is retreating massively year by year as a result of global warming. India has a grip on the flow to Bangladesh downstream with the Frakka Barrage, which is 10 km on the Indian side of the border. Until 1998, India used the Frakka Barrage to direct water to Calcutta in an attempt to prevent that port from drying up. However, this so seriously compromised Bangladeshi agriculture that the two countries eventually agreed to a more equitable arrangement. Nevertheless, water quality has deteriorated sharply because of the high levels of arsenic and untreated sewage in the Ganges.[20]

The water situation in Latin America

On 22 May 2006, I received the following email.

> Dear friends who care about our earth:
>
> Judge for yourself if you want to take action.
>
> In the Valle de San Felix, the purest water in Chile runs from two rivers, fed by two glaciers. Water is a most precious resource, and

wars will be fought for it. Indigenous farmers use the water, there is no unemployment, and they provide the second largest source of income for the area. Under the glaciers has been found a huge deposit of gold, silver and other minerals. To get these, it would be necessary to break, to destroy the glaciers – something never conceived of in the history of the world – and to make two huge holes, each as big as a whole mountain, one for extraction and one for the mine's rubbish tip.

The project is called PASCUA LAMA. The company is called Barrick Gold. The operation is planned by a multinational company, one of whose members is George Bush, Senior. The Chilean government has approved the project to start in 2006. The only reason it hasn't started yet is because the farmers have got a temporary stay of execution. If they destroy the glaciers, they will not just destroy the source of especially pure water, but they will permanently contaminate the two rivers so they will never again be fit for human or animal consumption because of the use of cyanide and sulphuric acid in the extraction process. Every last gram of gold will go abroad to the multinational company, and not one will be left with the people whose land it is. They will only be left with poisoned water and the resulting illnesses.

The farmers have been fighting a long time for their land, but have been forbidden to make a TV appeal by a ban from the Ministry of the Interior. Their only hope now of putting the brakes on this project is to get help from international justice. The world must know what is happening in Chile. The only place to start changing the world is from here.

Recipients were requested to circulate the message, with each 100th signatory sending it to mailto:noapascualama@yahoo.ca, to be forwarded to the Chilean government.

A bit of detective work traced the email to a Canadian group dedicated to changing public policy with regard to large-scale mining projects, and designed to protect the health of individuals, communities and entire ecosystems. The group claims that the Pascua Lama Project can be stopped – a very important point for us to keep in mind.

So far the Chilean National Environmental Commission (CONAMA) has accepted 42 of the 46 complaints filed against the government's own regional Environmental Commission (COBEMA). The reader will recall that, early in 2006, Michelle Bachelet was elected President in Chile, on a ticket that promised protection of the poor and of the environment, and the new head of CONAMA has strong green credentials.

The mining company, Barrick, has not said how it is going to mine without disturbing the already damaged glaciers. It certainly has not addressed the issue of water use and possible contamination on both sides of the Argentine–Chile border. In addition, the US$ 60 million deal, by which Barrick tried to buy off the opposition, has been declared invalid by the Public Works Ministry's General Directorate of Waters. The rights of the indigenous people affected are still being argued, and the case is due to go before the International Human Rights Commission.

As the reader is probably aware, the election of the first female president of Chile was remarkable in itself, but all the more so because Michelle Bachelet's family, who had been prominent in Chilean human rights agitation prior to the brutal Pinochet regime, had suffered extensively under that regime. Therefore Michelle Bachelet more than almost anyone else should understand the need to protect the human rights of indigenous people. However, she and her government will have the full weight of global financial pressure brought against them. It is here that a massive influx of letters from thousands of ordinary concerned people can make a decisive difference. After having come to power at least partly as an antidote to Pinochet's acquiescence to the neoliberal developed world banking interests, she would not want to lose face by siding with the same forces.

Chile is not alone among South American countries facing privatisation of their water supplies, or their water supply being compromised by various WTO-style bilateral agreements.

For instance, four Latin American countries – Argentina, Brazil, Bolivia and Paraguay – share the Guarani Aquifer. This has a volume of about 40,000 km^3 and is a crucial source of drinking water for all four countries. However, the US military base near the country's main airport has recently been making huge demands on this aquifer, and that has raised concerns.

Indeed a film was made, 'Sed, Invasiones Gota a Gota' ('Thirst, Invasions, Drop by Drop'), which featured the US activities in this regard. Particularly worrying is the presence of a large US military encampment on the common frontier between Paraguay, Argentina and Brazil. It was the ready supply of water that attracted the US developers to the region, and this has caused widespread fear that their projected use of it might threaten the livelihoods of hundreds of thousands of people. Such concerns have been very well articulated in newspaper articles,[21,22] and these worries have been heightened by a military agreement in 2005–06 between Paraguay and the USA, highlighted by a visit there by US Secretary of Defence Donald Rumsfeld. The latter was dealing not only with the Paraguayan government, but also with that of Bolivia. As the reader may remember, widespread unease among the Bolivian people about US exploitation of that country's gas resources was one factor that led, in December 2005, to the election of Evo Morales – a worrying development for US business interests. In fact Morales was not alone, once elected, in approaching Venezuela's Hugo Chavez about working out a joint policy on such issues. Is it any wonder that the USA called the events a 'factor of instability in the region'?

Present neoliberal methods mean that the only way available for LDCs to develop well enough to participate in 'free trade', as promoted by the WTO, is for them to create an infrastructure dominated by foreign-owned plants. These issues have brought water control to international attention, and have dramatically changed the relationship between people in many LDCs and their customary sources of water. The argument that water privatisation was a necessary part of 'development for free trade' was trenchantly put by David Green.[23] He pointed out that when Coca-Cola set up a bottling plant in India, its demand for water denied local farmers enough to sustain either their produce or their families. Green argued that this is the price that must be paid if a poor country wants to develop. The Indian government thought so, too (*see* Chapter 7), and readily accepted Coca-Cola's payment to disenfranchise their own citizens. In effect, what Green is saying is that the commercial advantage (if the payment is large enough) of some must prevail over the human rights of all.

In 1989, Margaret Thatcher, then Prime Minister of the UK, implemented a huge water privatisation scheme for the whole of England and Wales. Suddenly a precious natural resource was taken from English and Welsh people, sold off and privatised, and the people affected now had to pay the water companies. They had to pay not only for the provision of water, but also to make a profit for the shareholders of the companies and to pay high management salaries. Water bills doubled in less than 10 years, and this caused acute hardship for many people. During this period there were 50,000 disconnections, and water quality steadily deteriorated.[24]

Privatisation of water supplies

Thus, even in developed countries, the private sector regularly has a negative impact on health and other basic human rights. Although it is probably true that, in most developed nations, the electorate would strongly object if ready access to clean water was not virtually universal, with the blessing of the IMF and related agencies, this is now happening in a number of LDCs. The implications are obvious. Not only is there a risk that poor people will refuse to access water if they have to pay for it, because they cannot afford it, but, as the World Development Movement has amply demonstrated, even the private firms that provide the water have failed to adequately safeguard its potability.

Because of this, such privatisations have been legally contested on several occasions because of bad water quality, high prices, etc. In fact, water privatisation even in the UK has not turned out to be such a juicy enterprise for corporate money grabbers as was originally thought in the heady days of Thatcherism. Water reticulation systems are extremely expensive and constantly need expensive sections replaced. The London water supply is still making use of miles of piping that was installed in Victorian times, and the system now leaks prodigiously. However, in the mean time, major parts of one of the world's largest cities have been built over that piping. Replacement and repair will be incredibly expensive. The private water company concerned is still making enormous profits both for its directors, none of whom are paid less than the equivalent of US$ 1 million a year, and for its stockholders. However, if they were to undertake a proper full-scale repair, with all of the expensive interruption of city life that that would entail, either their profits would have to be slashed or their customers would have to pay astronomical water bills. They are truly stuck. Of course this is one reason why, if complex society is to be run fairly, government has to run such utilities, paying for them through taxation rather than by user payment. Water has to be easily accessible, at a small price to users.

In LDCs, water companies are beginning to realise this. In Bolivia, for example, the privatisation of water supplies proposed by the IMF as part of its structural adjustment caused such large price increases that there were serious riots in 2000 in Cochabamba. These caused Bechtel, an American water corporation based in San Francisco, to pull out from Bolivia. Another water company, SUEZ, has started to pull out of various South American countries after prolonged rioting and violence. Bolivian officials took SUEZ to task for failing to connect enough households to water supplies to meet its contractual obligations. It found itself having to charge up to US$ 55 per household. This was more than three times a lower-middle-class wage, according to *Mercury News*.[25]

Since water is a basic human right, and it is expensive to mediate the supply while not heavily charging individual consumers, there is simply no logical way of making a profit out of it. Like such public services as health and schooling, it is not a fit vehicle for private enterprise.

Dirty aid, dirty water: the WDM Campaign

As mentioned previously, the World Development Movement has taken a leading role in exposing details of water privatisation projects in LDCs, and in making their findings widely available on the Internet. The 'Dirty Aid' campaign has concentrated on the degree to which respected international aid agencies, both governmental and non-governmental, have been inveigled into supporting private enterprise in privatising water supplies, and the difficulties that the recipient countries have encountered in trying to extricate themselves from their contractual obligations if the quality of the water supply fails to satisfy health requirements. Of course, even some government-sponsored water supply systems, through corruption or other forms of malfeasance, have similarly failed to meet minimum health standards.

Because of such factors, many communities have been inspired to take the issue into their own hands – fighting corruption and incompetence to make efficient water systems accessible to even the poorest people in the community. To quote the WDM:

> UK policy on supporting access to water is a one-trick pony. The Department for Industry and Development (DfID) seems to be addicted to an approach that neglects community-based water reform options.[26]

In other words, the DfID seems almost perverse in its failure to learn from successful examples of local control of water supplies, and instead funding foreign private companies to do the job. This, of course, is entirely in keeping with IMF/World Bank policy – as far as the funding for the project is concerned – and also fits with the WTO/GATS policy in allowing such private firms to compete against local, community-based enterprises. While the DfID is throwing millions of pound at failed privatisation, it barely acknowledges community-based solutions.

This misuse of aid, of course, has its basic free market agendas, creating policies that serve corporate interests. The 'Dirty Aid, Dirty Water' campaign of the WDM seeks economic justice, allowing communities to make their own decisions and putting the rights of the people affected ahead of those of remote business interests. Since everyone should have ready access to clean water at little or no cost, the relevant infrastructure should be owned by government and funded through taxation.

A brief overview of the kinds of initiatives undertaken by WDM is provided by their 'case studies' accessible on the Internet (www.wdm.org.uk/campaigns). Ghana, the first of the African colonies to gain independence, was also the first to be considered by the WDM. Local companies there are vehement in their insistence that the hugely unpopular water privatisation they are fighting was in fact imposed upon their government by the World Bank, and strongly backed up by their former colonial masters, the UK. Not only that, but money from the UK that was destined for aid had been used to finance this failed solution to Ghana's water crisis.

Originally, the UK government had encouraged the private firm Biwater plc to bid for the project. After a targeted campaign by the WDM, Biwater eventually pulled out of the bidding. In Ghana, as everywhere else, access to safe water is vital to life. However, in Ghana almost half the population has no regular water supply. Obviously the most vulnerable – the elderly, the very young and the poor – are the most adversely affected by this situation. For instance, in the rural areas where most of Ghana's people live, two-thirds of the population regularly risk disease by using unclean water. Likewise, in the slum areas of the cities, sewage – if it is carried away at all – flows down trenches, and only about 10% of families have their own water supply system.

In a typical slum household in Accra (the capital of Ghana), 40 pence a day might be spent on water – about as much as a middle-class household in London! In Ghana, 40 pence is a day's earnings. Hawa Arnadu, a widow in her seventies, runs one such household and lives with three of her six surviving children. They have to travel nearly 2 km a day to fetch water. She was quoted as saying that she often goes without food so that the children can have water. Forcing Ghana to privatise its water supply has made an already dire situation even worse, and delays in implementing payment for a privatised supply have caused a rapid rise in waterborne diseases. All of this has stimulated grass-roots anger and violent disturbances.[27]

Sierra Leone is another country with very similar problems. It is just emerging from 10 years of civil war, and is ranked by the UN as the second poorest nation on earth. Only 28% of its population have access to adequate water and sanitation. However, it is the latest target for UK-based water privatisation. The WDM could find no evidence that alternative solutions were even considered.

Nevertheless, we can be encouraged by the knowledge that some WDM campaigns are working! In October 2005, as a direct result of WDM pressure, the UK's Department for Industry and Development (DfID) backed down on its intentions to use aid money to fund a huge public relations campaign promoting community support for the privatisation of Sierra Leone's public water supply. The DfID had decided instead to spend the money on a public communications and education programme. The deadline for the bid had originally been 20 October 2005. The DfID, after its change of heart, wrote to all the short-listed companies indicating that they should withdraw their bids.

The WDM's case study of Tanzania makes equally grim reading. In that country, 60% of the population live on less than US$ 2 per day, and 9.8 million Tanzanians have no access to safe water. As a result, about 40% of children under 5 years of age suffer from diarrhoea. Since 1991, the water supply in the capital, Dar es Salaam, had been pushed to privatise, but in May 2005, Tanzania called off its contract with Biwater. However, in June 2005 Biwater announced that its partner, City Water, had successfully applied to the court for 'an interim injunction' to prevent the Tanzanian government from unlawfully terminating the contract without submitting it to arbitration.[28] In other words, City Water is trying to secure compensation from the government of Tanzania! In December 2005, the

WDM discovered that Biwater was intent on going ahead and suing the cash-strapped and indebted Tanzanian government.[29]

WDM's Director, Benedict Southworth, said:

> This is an absolute disgrace. Tanzania is one of the poorest countries in the world, and now Tanzanian citizens are being punished for being the victims of a failed policy which they did not want. The privatisation, a condition of debt relief, seriously lacks legitimacy.[30]

According to the Tanzanian government, City Water failed to supply, with people on the ground reporting that water delivery was getting worse in many areas. In 2004, Action Aid International found that households that were unable to pay their water bills were summarily disconnected. Benedict Southworth described this as a 'bullying tactic.'[31] Furthermore, even the UK taxpayers end up paying Biwater's Tanzanian bills, because their contracts are insured with the UK Export Credit Guarantee Department (ECGD). In the mean time, some of the UK's 'aid' to Tanzania is being spent on the aggressive promotion of Biwater by TV and radio advertising and even pop songs. The Tanzanian Association of NGOs strongly endorses their government's action in dismissing Biwater.

Not all case studies put out by the WDM have recorded failures, of course. It has recorded as successful the public water schemes in Doha, Bangladesh, Kerala, India and Penang, and Malaysia, and some schemes in Brazil. However, among its more spectacular recordings of failure have been those in Tanzania, Trinidad, Guyana and Bolivia. In summary, we can say that the World Development Movement provides a fine example of what NGOs can accomplish in the area of human rights through persistent and public representation of abuses.

Impact of dams on human rights

It is of course obvious that water management does not only involve elaborating methods for supplying safe drinking water. It must include the ways in which existing supplies of water are harnessed for irrigation and for provision of power for electricity generation, etc. This raises the question of dam construction. There are at least 45,000 large dams operating around the world (as of July 2006), and a further 1,500 are currently under construction.[32] Dams, canals and other diversions interrupt the flow of 60% of major rivers globally. In fact some rivers, such as the Colorado, Rio Grande and Yellow River, no longer reach the sea at various times of year because fragmentation has led to significant decreases in water flow.[33]

However, it would be a mistake to assume that the construction of dams is a complete perversity. The problem is that the agencies that have the power and authority to construct dams often vastly underestimate the huge negative impact that such projects can have on the health and other human rights of thousands of people who have little or no political or economic influence. Dams are also the cause of extensive environmental damage and community upheaval.[34] A report based on analyses of 125 dams in the year 2000 by the World Commission on Dams (WCD) showed that ecosystem damage occurred in 67% of the cases checked, including destruction of fishing, accumulation of sewage, etc. For instance, damming the Danube River in Europe has caused two species of sturgeon to become extinct. A similar catalogue of economically important ecological setbacks has attended dam construction on the Yangtze River in China.

Of course, humans have not escaped these effects. According to the WCD, 40 to 80 million people worldwide have either lost their homes because of the building of dams, or have had to relocate because they can no longer sustain a livelihood due to the environmental destruction. A good example of this is the dam on the Tocantins River in Brazil. The dam, called Tucurai, reduced fish catches by 60%. Other dams in the same river have deprived farmers downstream of enough irrigation for them to be able to continue to make a living.[35]

In March 2006, the Latin American Water Tribunal in Mexico released its verdict from a public hearing that was held in order to consider the human rights violations brought about by the construction of the Multipurpose Dam Project in the Guayas River Basin in Ecuador. The opposing parties were the Coordinator of the Defence of Life and the Environment in the Guayas River Basin (CEDEGE) and the Food First International and Action Network (FIAN International). In opposition were three ministries of the Government of Ecuador (the Ministry of Government, the Ministry of the Environment and the Ministry of Health) and the State Studies Commission for the development of the Guayas River Basin.

At the hearings it emerged that the affected communities had not been consulted and no previous health impact assessment had been made, nor had there been any evaluation that anticipated the modifications of the river's dynamics, the deforestation, and soil erosion and social conflict due to water shortages. If people were compensated, this was not done adequately. The water quality has deteriorated and this has led to several outbreaks of waterborne infections. Local communities had requested an environmental assessment before building began, but this was ignored. Even two requests from the government's own Ministry of the Environment produced no action. Then, on 9 October 2004, the Ecuadorean Government ruled that the multipurpose dam project was a 'national priority', and all complaints against it were dismissed.

However, for the first time ever it was argued that, since access to safe and potable water is now a basic human right under the UN Charter, the dam represented a violation of human rights. The committee ruled that 'Drinking water of adequate quantity and quality is an elemental constituent of human dignity and a major component for the exercise of all other human rights.'[36] The outcome was that the Latin American Water Tribunal resolved to censor the Ecuadorean government and its state institutions for not fulfilling their duties of respecting, protecting and guaranteeing the human rights and basic needs of the inhabitants settled in the Guayas River Basin.[37]

Much more could be written on the issue of dam construction. One has only to think of now well-reported damming projects in India and China (the Three Gorges Dam). Suffice it to say that these problems grow worse by the day. They will continue to worsen unless radical changes are made which specfically link in with the satisfaction of human rights criteria, as vetted by internationally mediated health impact assessments. Indeed, the UN stressed the significance of the issue when it proposed 'Water for Life' as the theme for the International Decade for Action 2005–2015. This was one of the items opposed by the US representative to the UN, John Bolten.[38] That resolution emphasised that 'Water is critical for sustainable development, including environmental integrity and the eradication of poverty and hunger, and is indispensable for human health and well-being.'[39]

Pollution and other water issues

The theme of access to safe and potable water raises a huge array of human rights issues, many of which will be addressed in subsequent chapters. For instance, privatisation, as promoted by such WTO arrangements as GATS and its frequent link with problems raised by TRIPS, itself serves to promote corporate business interests ahead of health rights. As we have seen, this is the case not only in less developed nations but also even in the most advanced developed nations. However, before dealing with this issue more fully, it is instructive to consider the privatisation of water in China, something which, in its desperate drive to 'develop' and become an important player in free trade, China undertook too hastily.

Five south-eastern Asian countries in addition to China itself receive their water largely from the Mekong river. Rising in Tibet, this river flows through China's Yunan province, and then runs through Myanmar (Burma), Thailand, Laos, Cambodia and Vietnam. Problems began in 1966 when China built the Manwan Dam, which grossly interfered with the downstream water supplies, as well as causing costly flash floods. Moreover, China is scheduled to complete six more dams in the next few years, and the smaller countries that will be adversely affected by this have already complained. Not one of these dams has been subjected to a Health Impact Assessment (HIA). In a previous publication, this author recommended that International Health Impact Assessments should be required before such large structures affecting other countries can be undertaken.[40]

However, the Bretton Woods institutions blithely override health rights considerations by making such projects an integral part of their SAPs. For instance, in 2003 the Asian Development Bank recommended construction of a US\$ 43 billion electricity-generating system, including major Mekong dams in Burma, China, Laos and Cambodia. The Mekong river already has over 100 dams. Vietnam, at the end of the chain, now finds its water supply severely compromised. And the dams planned for Laos will displace nearly 6,000 people and have an adverse impact on the agricultural production sustaining 120,000 others who are already living marginally. Moreover, the electricity produced will not be going to those countries, but will be sold by China to Thailand!

The impact on China itself will be negative. Already the water table there is falling by 3 metres a year. In fact, He Quingcheng, Head of the Geological Monitoring Institute in Beijing, has warned that North-West China is running down its last water reserves,[41] and it is in that region that China grows most of its wheat for domestic consumption. However, as far as this author has been able to determine, none of the affected people or their representatives have appealed their government's decision on the basis of the UN's 2002 definition of access to water as a basic human right under the Charter.

References

1 General Comment 15 on the right to water; www.undhs.ch/html/mem2./6cescr.htm (accessed 29 May 2006).
2 Trimlett G. 'Save the planet – don't play golf!' *The Guardian*, 16 July 2004, p. 3.
3 De Stefano L. *The Coming Water Crisis.* WWF pamphlet. Godalming: World Wide Fund for Nature; 2004.

4 Craig N. *World Rescue: climate facts demand action*. London: Housemans Bookshop Publications; 2002. p. 7.

5 Craig N, op. cit., p. 10.

6 www.jtkeflairships.com (email advertisement received June 2006).

7 http://cyberschoolbus.un.org/student/2005/theme.asp (accessed 30 May 2006).

8 World Water Watch. *A Chronology of Water-Related Conflicts*; http://worldwater.org/conflict.htm (accessed 15 June 2006).

9 Wikipedia. *Water Consumption Indicated in OECD Countries*; www.environmental indicators.com/htdocs/indicators/6wate.htm (accessed 30 May 2006).

10 MacDonald T. *Health, Trade and Human Rights*. Oxford: Radcliffe Publishing; 2005. p. 52.

11 BBC World Service. *Ogallala Aquifer: water hotspots*. Broadcast 24 May 2006; http://news.bbc.co.uk/1/shared/spl/hi/world/03/world_forum/water/html (accessed 15 June 2006).

12 BBC World Service; http://news.bbc.co.uk/1/shared/spl/hi/world/03/world_forum/water/mexico_city.stm (accessed 31 May 2006).

13 BBC World Service. *Water Shortages Foster Terrorism*. Broadcast 17 March 2003. http://news.bbc.co.uk/1/hi/sci/tech/2859937.stm (accessed 18 March 2003).

14 *Major Aspects of Scarce Water Resources Management in Arab Countries*. International Conference on Water Politics in Arid Zones, 1–3 December 1999, Amman, Jordan; http://mondediplo.com/2000/02/05chesnot (accessed 31 May 2006).

15 Israel–Jordan Treaty of Peace. Annexe 11, article 11, para.1, p. 57.

16 Chesnot C. Drought in the Middle East. *Le Monde Diplomatique*, February 2000 issue, p. 4; www.monde-diplomatique.Fr./2000/02/CHESNOT/13213.html (accessed 15 June 2006).

17 Darwish A. *Analysis. Middle East Wars*. BBC World Service Broadcast, 30 May 2006; http://news.bbc.co.uk/2/hi/middle_east/2949768.stm (accessed 15 June 2006).

18 BBC World Service. *Israel: water hotspots*. Broadcast 6 June 2006; http://news.bbc.co.uk/1/shared/spl/hi/world forum water/Israel.stm (accessed 15 June 2006).

19 BBC World Service. *Turkey: water hotspots*. Broadcast 13 June 2006; http://news.bbc.co.uk./1/shared/spl/hi/world/03/world_forum/water/html/Israel.stm (accessed 15 June 2006).

20 BBC World Service. *Ganges river: water hotspots*. Broadcast 24 May 2006; http://news.bbc.co.uk/1/shared/spl/hi/world/03/world_forum/water/html/river_ganges.stm (accessed 15 June 2006).

21 International Relations Centre. *US Moves in Paraguay Rattle Regional Relations*; http://america,irc_onlin_org/am/2991 (accessed 15 June 2006).

22 Sanchez C. US Marines put a foot in Paraguay (editorial). *El Clarin*, 14 December 2005, p. 2.

23 Green D. *The Demand for Water and Privatisation*; www.issue.com?aid+563648ca=world+affairs (accessed 9 November 2006).

24 Mesbahli M. *Water Wars*; www.countercurrents.org/en_mesbahli251104.htm (accessed 15 June 2006).

25 Browne, ADL. Bolivia's water wars coming to an end under Morales. *Mercury News*, 25 February 2006, p. 6.

26 World Development Movement. *Dirty Aid, Dirty Water. Campaign summary*. London: World Development Movement; 2005. p. 1.

27 Ibid., p. 3.

28 World Development Movement. *Case Study: Tanzania*. London: World Development Movement; 2005.

29 Ibid., p. 2.

30 Ibid., p. 3.

31 Ibid., p. 3.

32 Rola AC. *Rivers at Risk:* towards a sustainable surface water resource management. www.sanrem.uga.edu/sanrem/database/pdf/LinkingResearch.pdf (accessed 19 January 2007).

33 Ibid., pp. 3–4.

34 Ibid., p. 4.

35 Ibid., p. 5.

36 Verdict from the Public Hearing, Mexico Latinoamerican Water Tribunal, March 2006. Published by the Literary Files of the University of Cuenca, Ecuador, May 2006.

37 Ibid., p. 12.

38 MacDonald T, op. cit., p. 122.

39 United Nations. *International Covenant on Economic, Social and Cultural Rights (CESR). Article 11 (The Right to an Adequate Standard of Living) and Article 12 (The Right to Health).* Brussels: United Nations Regional Information Centre for Western Europe; 2002.

40 MacDonald T, op. cit., p. 122.

41 Mesbahli M, op. cit., p. 6.

Chapter 5

Inequalities in global wealth distribution

Statement of the problem

Commentaries about wealth inequality are often replete with remarks such as '25% of the world's population live on less than US$ 1.00 per day' or 'The richest 10% of the population controls 50% of the wealth.' However, such observations often lack analytical rigour, and this makes it impossible to meaningfully compare nations globally. For instance, Cubans have much less disposable income than, say, Canadians, but are they less wealthy? The answer depends on how one measures wealth. In a socialist economy, the citizens do not pay most of the cost of things like schooling, medical care, housing, etc. These items certainly cost money, but most of the money does not come out of the income of individual citizens.

Looking at the situation globally, as is being attempted in this book, we have to try to address the problem of comparing the wealth of various groups in different societies. Usually various racial and ethnic groups possess different amounts of wealth. This is also true if we categorise people by, say, age, clinical health, years of formal education, gender, etc. One very common approach has been to compare the wealth of the top 10% of the population with that of the bottom 10%. The greater the wealth equity of a society, the closer these two measures will be. Governments that are intent on improving wealth equity can use a variety of procedures for doing so. In most First World societies, we tend to rely mainly on some kind of 'progressive taxation' to accomplish this goal.

Under this system, those whose wealth is below the 'average' pay a lower percentage of their income in tax, and also receive a greater share of government-funded 'wealth' in terms of healthcare, schooling, etc. People whose levels of wealth are above this 'average' have to pay a higher proportion of their income in tax, and thus have to pay more towards such benefits as healthcare and schooling. Another way of improving health equity would be to enforce greater equality by government diktat, so that a person's salary is not determined by normal free-market supply-on-demand economics, but by government directly.

There exists an enormous literature critical of both systems.

As the matter stands now (in 2006), most wealth is concentrated among the G8 nations (France, the USA, the UK, Italy, Germany, Japan, Canada and Russia). In fact, the G8 nations together with a number of Asian countries own over 70% of global wealth. Within individual nations among the G8, there is considerable variation. For example, in the USA, the wealthiest 1% of the population controls 38% of the wealth, while the bottom 40% own less than 1% of the wealth.[1]

Figure 5.1 makes the point rather effectively, using 2004 data. For obvious reasons, this type of presentation is often referred to as a 'champagne-glass' figure. Of course, we have to imagine a champagne glass with a hollow stem and, even more remarkably, no base!

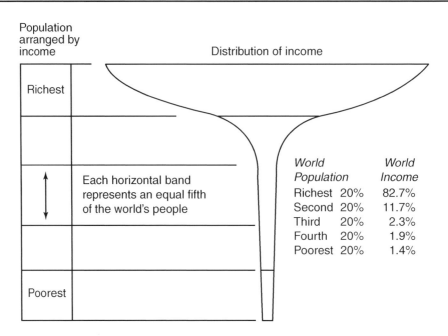

Figure 5.1 Champagne glass of income distribution.

As we have already seen, the world is a very unequal place, and this diagram shows an approximation of the income distribution of the world. The population of the world is divided into fifths, with the richest fifth having 83% of the world's income and the poorest fifth having 1.4% of it.[2] In the 1960s, the income of the wealthiest fifth was 30 times greater than that of the poorest fifth. It is now 80 times greater. As the world has become wealthier, the rich have got richer and the poor have either got poorer or stayed about the same.[3]

Wealth and income

What do we mean by 'wealth'? It is not the same as 'income.' The easiest way for the reader to understand it is to think of 'wealth' as being constant for a person or group. It is a fixed amount which, in part, is made up of the total of incomes (the plural is intentional) that the person or group has received up to that point. 'Income', on the other hand, is a fluctuating function. Figure 5.2 should make this clear.

This 'income' represents a 'rate of change', and hence its analysis must invoke an encounter with mathematical analysis. The author will endeavour to explain this encounter in reader-friendly terms. For a further explanation of these subtleties the reader is referred to the author's book on mathematical analysis for the lay reader.[4]

Measuring income inequality

Economists use various income distribution measures to describe levels of income inequality, either globally or within one country. As described by the author,[5] these measures are categorised as either 'absolute' or 'relative.' Briefly, 'absolute' measures define a minimum standard (often calculated differently by different countries). There are two very important measures of absolute income.

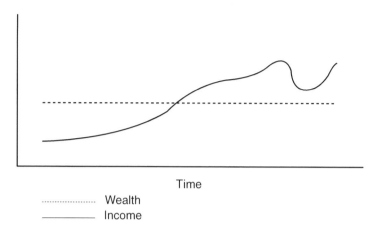

Time

·················· Wealth

———————— Income

Figure 5.2   Difference between wealth and income over a lifetime.

1 The *poverty line*. This is defined as the level of income necessary to subsist in a society. It will vary from one society to another, and over time within any one society, according to such criteria as cost of living and people's expectations. It is usually calculated as that level of income at which a household will use two-thirds (or three-quarters, in some cases) of its income on basic necessities (food, shelter and clothing).

2 The *poverty index*. This was defined by Amartya Sen[6] to take account of the number of poor people and the degree of their poverty. Sen defined the index by the simple algebraic formula:

$$I = \frac{\left(\dfrac{P}{N}\right)(B-A)}{A}$$

where P = number of people living below the poverty line, N = total number of people in the society, B = actual poverty line income and A = average income of these people living below the poverty line.

Relative income measures

The idea behind *relative* income measures is to allow comparison between individuals or even groups within the same population. They tend to be most useful when analysing the range and distribution of income inequality. Some examples that are useful in the context of this author's argument include the following:

- percentile distributions
- Lorenz curve
- Gini coefficient
- Robin Hood index.

To understand percentile distributions, the reader has to be clear about the difference between a percentage and a percentile. A *percentage* is a fraction of 100. Thus 3% of, say, 51,650 is 3 × 516 + 3 × ½ = 1,549.5, because there are 516 hundreds in 51,600 and half of a hundred in 50. A *percentile*, on the other hand, refers to rankings, from 0% to 100% of the list of numbers from the lowest to the highest. For instance, it might be calculated that the income of the top 10-percentile is only slightly in excess of the bottom 40-percentile. Thus percentile refers to an ascending number scale of 100 equal divisions of a range of statistical data (e.g. incomes), that indicates the value below which any given percentage of the data lies. For example, if a person (or community) is at the 83rd percentile on the income range, this means that 17% of the population concerned is above that income.

Another common division of percentile is the *quartile*, there being four quartiles. Thus one can come across a reference to, say, the top quartile having 45% of the society's total income, while the bottom quartile has only 10% of it. In this context, too, the reader will often come across references to the 'inter-quartile' range, which is the percentile range of 25% to 75%.

The Lorenz curve is a most useful device which the author will explain in sufficient detail later in this chapter to enable the reader to use it. For now, suffice it to say that it refers to a graph which is used to display the relative inequality in a given distribution of income values. Basically, a society's total income is ordered according to income level, and then the *cumulative total* (the sum up to the point to which one is referring) is graphed.

The Gini coefficient is a statistic used to quantify the extent of income inequality shown on a given Lorenz curve. The deeper meaning of this will become clear to the reader shortly! For now, though, let us set *absolute* and *relative* incomes in context.

Both are used as a basis for evaluating poverty. However, as implied earlier, income does not only refer to money. If a poor subsistence farmer grows, say, half of their own food from seeds gained with a cash transfer, it still counts as 'income.' Even more abstractly, as mentioned with regard to Cuba, services such as primary healthcare, milk supplements and schooling provided at no direct cost to the consumer count as income. These things are notoriously difficult to quantify. For instance, the World Bank uses the Living Standard Measurement Survey (LSMS)[7] to measure income. This involves completing a questionnaire containing over 200 items, and surveys have been undertaken using this instrument in most First World countries. The reader can appreciate the operational difficulties in trying to use the LSMS in developing countries with high rates of illiteracy and low levels of education!

The Lorenz curve explained

The Lorenz curve is a graph that shows, for the lowest *x*% of households (the abscissa measure on the graph), what percentage the corresponding *y*% (the ordinate measure on the graph) of the population have.

In the population shown in Figure 5.3, the increases are very unfairly distributed. For instance, 50% of the households account for only 40% of the income! Even 80% of the households still account for much less than 80% of the income, as can be seen on the graph. On the other hand, the broken straight line, running at a 45° angle to the *x*-axis and having a positive slope, would represent a perfectly fair distribution, because the more the curve deviates from the straight line of slope +1, the less fair the distribution is.

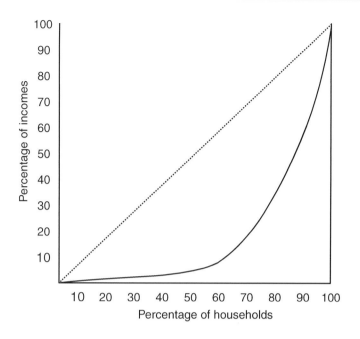

Figure 5.3 A Lorenz curve of income distribution of a hypothetical population.

It was Max O Lorenz, a US economist, who developed the curve that takes his name, in 1905. Corrado Gini, an Italian statistician, carried Lorenz's work just a little further to give us the Gini coefficient, which allows us to make better analytical comparisons. The Gini coefficient is a vital tool for discussing human rights, and it is important to at least appreciate how it works.

To understand it, the reader needs to have a basic insight into probability theory as applied to statistical inference. An accessible account of this is given by the author in his publication on epidemiological analysis for healthcare workers.[8]

The Gini coefficient

Originally intended to systematise and more rigorously quantify Lorenz's analysis of unequal income distributions, the Gini coefficient can be used to analyse any form of uneven distribution. The Gini coefficient is a number between 0 and 1, where 0 corresponds to 'perfect equality.' In other words, it allows us to calculate a measure of the degree to which a distribution deviates from the 'perfect', which is represented by the broken line in Figure 5.3.

Now let us look at Figure 5.4.

In a state of perfect equality, the Gini coefficient would equal 0, and in a state of complete inequality where one person in the community in the population had all the income, the Gini coefficient would equal 1. Figure 5.4 represents neither of these. But how does one calculate the Gini coefficient?

Notice that in Figure 5.4 we have designated the area between the Lorenz curve and the perfect equality line as A. Likewise, the area between the *x*-axis (abscissa) and the Lorenz curve is designated B. The Gini coefficient, G, is then given by the formula:

$$G = \frac{A}{A+B}$$

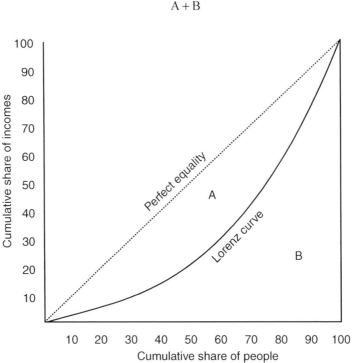

Figure 5.4 Graph for calculating a Gini coefficient

The reader will find that, in some publications, the G-score is multiplied by 100, so those scores can range from 0 to 100 instead of from 0 to 1. Although no hard and fast rule prevails, this practice seems to be increasing.

Using this formula will introduce a slight inaccuracy because of some rather involved statistical phenomena, which control variance, arising when using the formula characteristics of G. However, this problem is overcome by multiplying the value you get for G by the fraction $n/n+1$, where n is the number of individuals (or communities) used.

Calculation of the areas A and B does require integral calculus. However, a more practical formula is given by:

$$G = 1 - \sum_{K=1}^{n} (X_K - X_{K=1}) \, (Y_K + Y_{K-1})$$

The use of the capital Greek letter Σ, called 'sigma', means the summing up of the areas of all the 'rectangles', each represented by each particular value of

$$(X_K - X_{K=1}) \, (Y_K + Y_{K-1})$$

for any given value of K. Sigma notation used in such calculations is explained fully in the author's book, *Foundations of Mathematical Analysis*.[9] Remember, though, that in some presentations the Gini score is multiplied by 100, so that the scores range from 0 to 100 instead of from 0 to 1.

Gini coefficients worldwide

Tables 5.1 and 5.2 show how Gini indices allow us to compare countries by income inequality.[8] These values are derived from *Gap Between Rich and Poor: World Income Inequality*.[10]

Table 5.1   The 30 countries with the greatest inequality

	Country	Gini index	Lowest 20%	Highest 20%
1	Sierra Leone	62.9	1.1	63.4
2	Central African Republic	61.3	2.0	65.0
3	Swaziland	60.9	2.7	64.4
4	Brazil	60.7	2.2	64.1
5	Nicaragua	60.3	2.3	63.6
6	South Africa	59.3	2.9	64.8
7	Paraguay	57.7	1.9	60.7
8	Colombia	57.1	3.0	60.9
9	Chile	56.7	3.3	61.0
10	Honduras	56.3	2.2	59.4
11	Guinea-Bissau	56.2	2.1	58.9
12	Lesotho	56.0	2.8	60.1
13	Guatemala	55.8	3.8	60.6
14	Burkina Faso	55.1	4.6	60.4
15	Mexico	53.1	3.5	57.4
16	Zambia	52.6	3.3	56.6
17	Hong Kong, China	52.2	4.4	57.1
18	El Salvador	52.2	3.3	56.4
19	Papua New Guinea	50.9	4.5	56.5
20	Nigeria	50.6	4.4	55.7
21	Mali	50.5	4.6	56.2
22	Niger	50.5	2.6	53.3
23	Gambia	50.2	4.0	55.3
24	Zimbabwe	50.1	4.7	56.7
25	Venezuela	49.5	3.0	53.2
26	Malaysia	49.2	4.4	54.3
27	Russia	48.7	4.4	53.7
28	Panama	48.5	3.6	52.8
29	Cameroon	47.7	4.6	53.1
30	Dominican Republic	47.4	5.1	53.3

Table 5.2   The 30 countries with the greatest equality

	Country	Gini index	Lowest 20%	Highest 20%
1	Slovakia	19.5	11.9	31.4
2	Belarus	21.7	11.4	33.3

Table 5.2 (Continued)

	Country	Gini index	Lowest 20%	Highest 20%
3	Hungary	24.4	10.0	34.4
4	Denmark	27.4	9.6	34.5
5	Japan	24.9	10.6	35.7
6	Sweden	25.0	9.6	34.5
7	Czech Republic	25.4	10.3	35.9
8	Finland	25.6	10.0	35.8
9	Norway	25.8	9.7	35.8
10	Bulgaria	26.4	10.1	36.8
11	Luxembourg	26.9	9.4	36.5
12	Italy	27.3	8.7	36.3
13	Slovenia	28.4	9.1	37.7
14	Belgium	28.7	5.3	37.3
15	Egypt	28.9	9.8	39.0
16	Rwanda	28.9	9.7	39.1
17	Croatia	29.0	8.8	38.0
18	Ukraine	29.0	8.8	37.8
19	Germany	39.0	8.2	38.5
20	Austria	31.0	6.9	38.0
21	Romania	31.1	8.0	39.5
22	Pakistan	31.2	9.5	41.1
23	Canada	31.5	7.5	39.3
24	Korea, South	31.6	7.5	39.3
25	Poland	31.6	7.8	39.7
26	Indonesia	31.7	9.0	41.1
27	Latvia	32.4	7.6	40.3
28	Lithuania	32.4	7.8	40.3
29	Spain	32.5	7.5	40.3
30	Netherlands	32.5	7.3	40.1

From Tables 5.1 and 5.2 the reader can see immediately the difference between the developed and less developed countries. For, instance, most European nations have Gini coefficients ranging between 0.24 and 0.36. The USA is markedly further away from income equality, and since 1985 its Gini coefficient has been above 0.4. Using this approach, human rights activists and scholars can quantify the debate with regard to welfare policies. However, as we shall see later, the Gini coefficient can lead us astray if we try to use it to make glib political comparisons between large and much smaller countries (e.g. between the USA and Cuba). Let us consider, for example, Hungary and Denmark. These two countries have the lowest Gini values in the EU. They were calculated separately in drawing up Tables 5.1 and 5.2. However, in the case of the USA, all of the states are (of course) calculated together, despite the fact that California, say, is extraordinarily rich, while some of the US states rate with less developed countries. If the value for each US state is calculated separately, their Gini score will generally be lower than that calculated for the country as a whole.

In the USA, as elsewhere, we see considerable variations in Gini scores over time (*see* Table 5.3).

Table 5.3   Changes in Gini score for the USA over 30 years

Year	Gini score
1970	0.394
1980	0.403
1990	0.428
2000	0.462

However, we note that the score is increasing, which suggests greater internal inequity.

Strengths of the Gini score as a measure of income inequality

1 Measures such as the gross domestic product (GDP) are not suitable for inter-country comparison because GDP is skewed by extreme values, which means that a GDP may well be very unrepresentative of most people in the country. The Gini score has a big advantage because it measures degrees of inequality, rather than an average.
2 The Gini score can be compared across countries and is easy to interpret. By comparison, GDP calculations are cumbersome and insensitive to variations across a given population.
3 We can use Gini scores to compare income distributions between various communities in a national population. As we would expect, for instance, Gini scores usually differ markedly between urban and rural areas within one country. When extremes of wealth and poverty are widely characteristic of both urban and rural subpopulations (as in the USA), the rural and urban Gini scores will remain close.
4 Because Gini scores seem to vary over time, they are useful for indicating how income distribution has changed over time in any one country.
5 Gini scores are independent of the size of the economy being measured. The same is true for differences in population size.

Critical comments on the use of the Gini score

1 As we have already seen in the case of the USA, if we use the Gini coefficient over a geographically large and diverse nation it will tend to result in a larger score than if the scores for the sub-regions are calculated individually. This makes it rather meaningless to compare, for example, the Gini scores of individual EU nations with that of the USA a whole.
2 Comparing incomes in different countries on the basis of Gini scores is problematic because different countries can have widely different welfare systems. For instance, a nation which provides housing and/or food stamps to its less fortunate citizens will have a higher Gini score than some nations which do not, because vouchers do not count as income when using the Gini coefficient.

3 Even if two nations have the same Gini coefficient, they may still differ greatly with regard to income distribution. For instance, suppose that in nation A half of the households had no income and the other half shared the entire income equally. This nation would have a Gini coefficient of 0.5. But so would nation B, in which the dictator has the entire nation's income and everyone else is equal – with no income at all!

4 Statistically speaking, the Gini coefficient responds more sensitively to incomes in the middle of the range than to incomes at the extremes.

These problems, especially the last one, have led to extra tests or variations on the Gini coefficient being elaborated. One of these is the Hoover index, also known as the Robin Hood index. It is equal to that portion of the total income that would have to be redistributed for there to be perfect equality. The reader can think of it as the longest vertical distance between the Lorenz curve (which, remember, is the cumulative portion of the total income held below a certain income percentile, and the straight line of slope +1). Hoover indices are often used for establishing links, within a society, between socio-economic status (SES) and health.

Another measure that is commonly referred to is the Atkinson index. It is one of the few that are actually biased, intentionally, towards the poorer end of the spectrum, so that it can be used when making judgements about the efficacy or otherwise of welfare programmes. It is derived by calculating what Atkins called the 'equity-sensitive average income', designated 'ye', which is defined as that level of per-capita income which – if enjoyed by everyone – would bring about total welfare equal to the total welfare generated by actual income distribution. The calculation of 'ye' is complex because it involves the calculation of a so-called 'inequality aversion parameter' or 'E', which requires rather esoteric mathematics. However, those details are not necessary for the reader to appreciate the argument. E reflects the strength of a society's preference for equality, and can take values ranging from zero to infinity. When E is greater than 0, there is a social preference for equality. As E increases in value, society attaches more weight to income transfers at the lower end of the distribution, while attaching less weight to such transfers at the upper end of the distribution.

The actual Atkinson index[1] is given by the formula:

$$I = 1 - \frac{ye}{m}$$

where m is the mean income of the population. The more equal the income generation, the closer 'ye' will be to m, and thus the lower the Atkinson index will be. Values of I range between 0 and 1.

There are other refinements of Gini, but it has been shown that the measures are all highly correlated with each other.[11]

The Marshall Plan revisited

In Chapter 2, the reader will recall, the role of the Marshall Plan as an aid programme in the reconstruction of post-war Europe was discussed. In that context, we saw it as a counterbalance to the rigid strictures of the IMF SAPs. Now let us consider it in the broader context of inequalities in global wealth distribution and of developed world control of less developed economies. In this chapter we have concerned ourselves with the issue of the vast disparities in wealth that characterise developed and less developed countries. Hegemonies of empires have always exercised their power through access to greater stores of wealth, and in this respect the US financial hegemony is no different. Yet how did it gain such powerful leverage, and so suddenly, after the Second World War? There are many reasons, but the Marshall Plan played a pivotal role in establishing it. A good spin was put on the Marshall Plan in the post-war years, and in many people's minds it still stands out as an example of the generosity of the wealthy USA towards those less fortunate countries. Even among groups that are highly critical of the role of the USA and the UK in Iraq, Afghanistan and elsewhere, the Marshall Plan brings back fond memories of a former time when US foreign policy seemed to be dominated by benevolence. Let us examine it a little more closely in order to understand how neoliberal global financial control really works.

The year 1945 saw the USA triumphant in war and in peace. The only thing that really stood between it and global financial domination was the USSR, along with the threat of communism spreading in other cultures worldwide. Domestically and overseas, US propaganda was intent on 'defeating communism', and the Marshall Plan was a carefully calculated part of that plan. It was regarded as crucial in opposing post-war tendencies in Greece, and even Italy and France, to adopt communist or socialist programmes, both as a means of post-war recovery and, more generally, as a means of removing the causes of war. Behind the Marshall Plan lay the realisation that US financial dominance required the opening of new markets for US corporations, encouraging the formation of the European Common Market and, of course, of NATO. This programme also called for a frontal attack on all communist and socialist organisations in universities, the media and elsewhere, and some Marshall Plan funds were used explicitly for such purposes. At the time, on the left, it was widely appreciated that US aid for France and Italy would be cut off if those countries did not take steps to counter domestic communism.

Before a country could receive money from the Marshall Plan, it had to agree to a series of economic and social criteria designed to promote free enterprise and its link with US corporate interests. This included such inducements as Fulbright and Ford foundation scholarships, and so on. In fact, US agencies had the right not only to say how Marshall Plan money was to be spent, but also to approve use of an equal amount of local currency. This gave US corporations a large degree of control over the economic policies of recipient nations. Moreover, a large proportion of Marshall Plan aid soon returned to the USA, as reconstruction programmes required the use of US goods and services.

Rather than the Marshall Plan being a fine example of open-handed charity, it can be seen – especially in retrospect – as exemplifying an effective partnership between US banks (and other corporations) and the ruling elites of European nations. In this way the Marshall Plan established the context from which developed what President Dwight Eisenhower, in an astonishing display of candour, called 'the military–industrial complex.'[12]

If one takes the time to study these issues closely, the 'open-handed charity' scenario does not stand up. There were 16 principal recipient nations. Without the overwhelmingly complete dispersal of Nazi power by the USA and the USSR, the USA would never have been in a position to take financial advantage of the situation. Without that distraction, indigenous economists for each of the 16 countries would have no doubt elaborated their own recovery plans, many of them socialist. Some of them had already taken significant steps along these lines before the inducement of the Marshall Plan funding made their governments decide otherwise.[13] The primary purpose of the Marshall Plan was to strengthen the economic infrastructure of heavy industry and power generators. In the countries concerned, these years were characterised by deflationary policies, recession and high unemployment. This was not charity, but the establishment of the basis for US global financial hegemony, in many respects an obstacle to human rights and the values of the UN Charter.

In Chapter 6 we shall analyse this further, first by giving some indication of the persistence of severely degrading poverty, and also by discussing its link to those transnational global interests that were given such impetus under initiatives like the Marshall Plan.

References

1 www.fairenonomy.org/research/wealth_charts.html (accessed 11 June 2006).
2 Gordon D. *Eradicating Poverty in the Twenty-First Century: when will social justice be done?* Inaugural Lecture at University of Bristol, delivered at the Townsend Centre for Industrial Poverty Research, Bristol. 18 October, 2004. p. 6 (text available from Bristol University Library).
3 Gordon D. Poverty, death and disease. In: Hillyard P, Pantazis C, Tombs S, Gordon D, editors. *Beyond Criminology: taking harm seriously.* London: Pluto; 2004. pp. 251–66.
4 MacDonald T. *Foundations of Mathematical Analysis: a journey of discovery for the layman.* Delhi: Ajanta Books; 2005. p. 413.
5 MacDonald T. *Third World Health: hostage to First World wealth.* Oxford: Radcliffe Publishing; 2005. pp. 93–108.
6 Sen A. Health and development. *Bull World Health Assoc.* 1999; **77:** 69–73.
7 www.worldbank.org/Isms (accessed 11 June 2006).
8 MacDonald T. *Basics of Statistics and Epidemiology for Health Workers.* Oxford: Radcliffe Publishing; 2006.
9 MacDonald T (2007) *Basic Concepts in Statistics and Epidemiology.* Oxford: Radcliffe Publishing.
10 World Bank. *Gap Between Rich and Poor: World Income Inequality. UN Human Development Index 2006.* Washington, DC: World Bank; 2006. pp. 315–16. www.infoplease.com/ipa/AD778562 (accessed 10 November 2006).
11 Kairachi I, Kennedy B. The relationship of income inequality to mortality. *Soc Sci Med.* 1997; **45:** 1121–7.
12 Eisenhower D. Military-Industrial Complex Speech; http://coursesa,matrix.msu.edu/2hst306/documents/indust.html (accessed 11 June 2006).
13 Kolko G, Kolko J. *The Limits of Power: the world and US foreign policy.* New York: Harper & Row; 1992. Chapters 13, 16 and 17.

Chapter 6

Poverty and primary healthcare

Poverty and health

Most people know, in a casual sort of way, that ill health and poverty are associated. However, in 1995 the World Health Organization stated that extreme poverty was the most serious cause of disease.[1] The same source goes on to say that 7 out of every 10 deaths in the less developed countries (LDCs) can be attributed to just five causes, namely pneumonia, diarrhoea, measles, malaria and malnutrition. We have the means to prevent virtually all such deaths, cheaply and easily. Pneumonia can be treated with the less expensive anti-biotics, diarrhoea can be arrested with standard saline–sugar packs at a penny a day, and measles is preventable by inoculation. Malaria has not yet attracted sufficient long-term financial interest for a cure to be available, but it can certainly be largely prevented by the use of bed-nets, and in a world characterised by massive overproduction (and then destruction) of food mountains, malnutrition is nothing less than an obscenity.

As the reader will be aware, most of the foregoing has been known or suspected for a long time. A few quotes indicate just how long we have been chewing this rag, but doing very little about it. US President Harry S Truman stated in his inaugural address in 1949:

> More than half of the people in the world are living in ... misery. Their food is inadequate. They are victims of disease ... their poverty is a threat to them and to more prosperous areas. But ... for the first time in history, humanity possesses the knowledge and skill to relieve the suffering of these people.[2]

However, we never got around to doing it, but 25 years later we were encouraged by none other than Henry Kissinger, who boldly stated in 1974 that 'Within a decade no child will go to bed hungry ... and no human being's future will be stinted by malnutrition.'[3]

In the 30 odd years since, we have not lacked for similar lofty assurances from various powerful people. We have had promises made and policies adopted by successive G7/G8 meetings, the issue has generated riots and demonstrations, and oceans of print have been used up in books (like this one). Our own New Labour government has been positively brimming over with anger at the delays, with Gordon Brown proclaiming in 2005 that 'In 2000 the world came together to make a solemn commitment to the Millennium Development Goals.'[4]

He then went on to point out that:

- universal primary education will be at least 115 years late
- halving global poverty will be at least 135 years late
- reduction in infant deaths will be 150 years late.

However, neoliberal financial orthodoxies, which are supported by all of the developed countries, and certainly by the UK and the USA, are having the opposite effect. The discrepancies between the developed countries and the LDCs are increasing, and it is often US scholars who are at the forefront in pointing this out.

Lifespan pyramids

For some time now, *lifespan pyramids* have been used to make the point, as is shown in Figures 6.1 and 6.2, which illustrate lifespan pyramids for an LDC, namely the Philippines, and for the USA – both using 1997 data.[5] The great advantage of such diagrams is that, at a glance, they give one a grasp of the most vulnerable points of the different parts of the life cycle, allowing one to identify periods of particular upheaval, such as wars or natural disasters in a nation's history. In the same way, they also show up baby booms. For instance, the Philippines is a much poorer country than the USA, and its death rate from birth onwards is higher. Over half the population will have perished by the age of 30 years. The Philippines chart also shows a high growth rate. In contrast, the lifespan pyramid for the USA reflects the more widespread availability of primary healthcare. The infant death rate is not seriously out of kilter with the death rate of all but the elderly. There is a definite bulge in population between the ages of 35 and 50 years, which reflects the post-war baby boom.

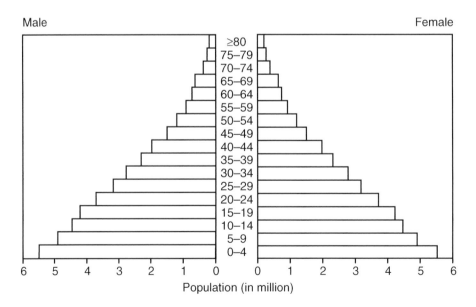

Figure 6.1 Lifespan pyramid for the Philippines, 1997. *Source:* US Census Bureau, International Database.

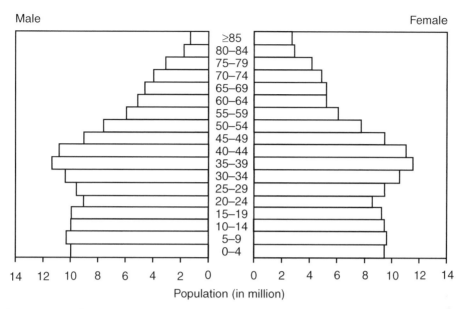

Figure 6.2 Lifespan pyramid for the USA, 1997. *Source:* US Census Bureau, International Database.

Factors that impoverish the LDCs

There are a number of developed world activities which, by impoverishing the LDCs, greatly increase child death rates – and indeed death rates for all age groups – in these countries. Reference has already been made to several of these activities. Race, and gender discrimination within race, play a large role. Loss of agricultural income within LDCs due to the impact of foreign agricultural products at lower prices under WTO–GATS provisions, and the use by developed-world firms of working conditions in the LDCs that would violate health and safety regulations in the home country are just two examples. While the need to restrict this book to a reasonable size limits the author in his coverage of these abuses, general reference will be made to illustrate the link to developed-world business interests and neoliberal financial orthodoxies.

This is important because the media that show interest in the rich world (e.g. Fox News, the various outreaches of the Murdoch Press, and even the British Broadcasting Corporation) have in the past been assiduous in their praise and support of 'freedom-fighting heroes' such as Lech Walesa, Andrei Sakharov and Vaclav Havel, who bravely opposed totalitarian regimes under previous Soviet control. Such coverage has led many people – especially in the non-communist world – to assume two things:

1 that systems which are practised and promoted in the anti-communist west must be free of those faults
2 that neoliberal finance must embody the antithesis of exploitation.

This is far from true. If any of the heroic figures mentioned above had been citizens of, say, El Salvador, they would have been quickly done away with by the death squads, which were equipped and even paid for by US corporate interests. The victory of the neoliberal democracies in the cold war has not, on the whole, been good news for the LDCs. Instead, it has led to a strengthening of powerful industrial countries, and has increased their capacity to throttle domestic economic development in poorer countries.

In 1992, Jack Nelson-Pallmeyer produced a well-documented book in which he points out that the new world order, based on neoliberal finance, is sustained by two 'police forces' – a military one and a financial one.[6] He refers to these as the two 'global cops', with the US military constituting the first (along with the UK and others), and the IMF and the World Bank, working through the WTO, representing the second. Furthermore, the power of these 'global cops' has been growing since the end of the Second World War, but at an accelerated rate since the oil crisis in the early 1990s.

Readers living in the developed world would view such a description as facile and superficial. However, when one lives and works in the poorer world, one finds that Nelson-Pallmeyer's analogy is deeply resonant among thinking people. The poor in the LDCs can justifiably argue that a primary reason for their plight is that they are victims of structural violence and injustice both at the hands of foreign multinational interests and at the hands of corrupt leaders in their own countries working as the clients of developed-world interests. In fact it is not difficult to see that most leaders of LDCs administer their economies, and their workforces, so as to enhance their own power. The effect is that under developed-world financial control, wealth is being transferred from the already poor LDCs to the developed world. There are many examples of this, but consider the extent to which the LDCs actually provide financial help with healthcare in the developed countries at the cost of their own.

Health aid flowing the wrong way

In the UK, if one has to undergo medical treatment at, say, a London hospital, one quickly appreciates the degree to which the NHS depends on overseas staff. One is attended by armies of Philippine nurses, doctors and medical technicians, to say nothing of the huge input from African countries and other parts of the less developed world. The NHS has not had to pay a penny for their excellent training. How great a difference has this made? Let us consider Figure 6.3.[7]

The UK's NHS began actively recruiting doctors and nurses from LDCs in December 2001 because they had calculated that by 2004 they would need 8,000–10,000 more doctors, and a far greater number of nurses than that, by 2004. That policy was stopped, as a matter of principle, a short time later, and this has made some difference. It is true that teams of NHS recruiting agents brandishing contracts were certainly a 'pull' factor. Corruption, inadequate facilities, lack of job security, low pay and discouragingly low standards of hospital hygiene in many LDCs acted as 'push' factors.

In addition, the NHS may have stopped actively recruiting, but private agencies have not. Between 1998 and 2004, shortages of hospital staff in the NHS hospitals were growing more acute, and many NHS facilities made use of private-agency staff, whom they had to pay at higher hourly rates than full-time staff. This represented an outrageous waste of NHS money and if any agency nurse then applied to join the NHS,without being explicitly recruited, it would not compromise the NHS's moral position if they agreed. As we shall see, this 'brain drain' of medical expertise from the LDCs to the much wealthier countries would have an immense impact on human rights issues.

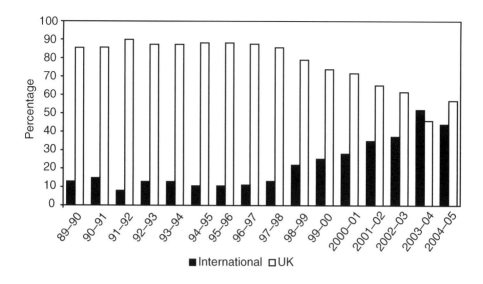

Figure 6.3 International and UK sources as a percentage of total new nurses admitted to the UK Register, 1989–90 to 2002–03 (initial registrations). *Source:* UKCC/NMC data.

However, cutbacks in NHS spending became necessary in late 2005, as more and more NHS trusts went into the red. This in itself was brought about by inroads of neoliberal finance pressure, to which the UK government of the time acquiesced. However, in 2006 the NHS found itself with a large number of overseas doctors who had been accepted to work in the NHS a year or so earlier, and who were now already registered in postgraduate specialist studies from which they had every intention of moving up the NHS consultancy hierarchy. Suddenly the NHS had to tell them that not only would they not receive funding to complete their studies, but also they were no longer needed in the NHS! It was all part of a cut-back routine.

The UK is not the only developed-world economy to be running into problems with financing healthcare, and one can foresee that many healthcare workers from LDCs will find themselves dislocated. For this reason, we need to look more broadly to developed countries' exploitation of medical and technical human resources trained in the LDCs. In 2001, South Africa actually requested Canada to stop poaching its newly qualified doctors, a strategy that was being adopted by Canada to fill gaps in its rural medical outreach. However, South Africa itself had already recruited 350 Cuban doctors to cover for the number of South African doctors who had taken up posts in the EU and North America.[8]

In the USA, 23% of doctors have qualified abroad, and in the UK about 20% of doctors are Asian in origin. In France 8,000 doctors have trained abroad, 4,000 of them outside Europe. Many of these are on night call, working in night wards and on children's and maternity wards, and in X-ray departments of state-run hospitals, but they do not qualify for the same conditions or salaries as their French colleagues. The developed world not only saves money by not paying for the expensive training, but also saves it on salaries! The Gulf States employ 20,000 doctors, mostly from the Indian subcontinent, although such south–south migration is usually temporary.

This talent drain has serious consequences. By the year 2000, only 360 of 1,200 doctors who had been trained in Zimbabwe in the 1990s were still working there. Half of the doctors who qualified in Ethiopia, Ghana and Zambia have left home, and many of them no longer work in medicine in their home country. The available statistics on voluntary migrants and refugees, and nationals born abroad, are not detailed enough to give an accurate picture of migratory movements.

The shortage of nurses was even more acute. In 2000, the UK added more than 8,000 nurses and midwives from outside the EU to the 30,000 overseas nurses already working in the state and private hospitals. Forecasts for the USA, France and the UK predict a shortfall of tens of thousands of qualified staff by the year 2010.

As of 2000, Sweden, which has an internationally recognised healthcare system, had to recruit 30 doctors trained in Poland. In the USA, 23% of the doctors had qualified in LDCs, and in the UK approximately 20% of the doctors registered in the year 2000 had qualified in Asian countries. In France, in 2002 the figure for doctors trained abroad was 8,000, of whom 4,400 came from the LDCs. Of course there is a historical context for all of this.[9]

We need to go back to Louis Pasteur (1822–1895). His discoveries revolutionised medicine and this had a great impact on the tropical colonies of European countries. Christian missionary activity alone accounted for a large transfer of medical expertise and of doctors from the developed world to less developed countries. Research-based medical advances over the next 30 years created increasingly extravagant expectations of good medical care by developed-world professionals. The demand for ever more doctors had outstripped domestic supply by the 1970s and, especially after the large-scale independence movement in the former African colonies, the flow of medical workers changed direction.[10]

As we have seen, the WHO's 'Health for All' initiative led that body to set health targets for LDCs. The aim was to provide one doctor for every 5,000 people and a qualified nurse for every 1,000 people. However, market forces, especially those promoted and guided by the Bretton Woods institutions, inevitably led to the abandonment of these aims. The world *average* is now one doctor for every 4,000 people, but there is no equity in the distribution, there being one for every 500 people in the developed world and one for every 25,000 people in the less developed world! India falls between these two extremes, with one for every 2,500 people.[11]

Consequences of inequity in primary healthcare

We must now direct our attention to the consequences of the decline in global equity with regard to the availability of primary healthcare. Not unnaturally, the international bodies responsible for deciding policy on health and fighting social inequality have little to say about this. Since 1979, neither the WHO nor the United Nations Development Program (UNDP) has published reports on the consequences of this trend for deprived populations.

The World Bank has published many studies celebrating the benefits of free markets, but it has not assessed the flow of funds resulting from exchanges of human capital. It no doubt prefers to disregard UN Resolution 2417 on the 'outflow of trained professional and technical personnel from the developing countries', which bans poaching of specialist professionals. It should be noted that a country's health service does not contribute directly to its gross domestic product.

In 1995, the WHO published a document entitled *Health for All in the Twenty-First Century*, which focused on the resources required for a global health policy. However, it made no attempt to control the movement of medical skills.[12] Nor does the WHO take account of missing doctors and nurses when calculating average lost years of good health, an index that factors in premature death and disability. Nor does the UNDP take the 'brain drain' into account in its human development index for each country. It may be impossible to quantify the suffering of people deprived of healthcare, but it is extremely clear why infant and maternal mortality has stopped declining. However, increasing public outcry about these inequities has had an effect. The WHO Director General has set up a commission on macroeconomics to propose a new approach to investment.

Their commission challenges the usual argument that health inevitably improves economic growth, stressing rather that improved health is essential to development and social progress in low-income countries. It calls for a new pact with regard to health to redefine relations between donor and beneficiary countries. However, it scarcely mentions the medical staff required to put such proposals into practice. In order to achieve its objectives, the global fund to fight AIDS, tuberculosis and malaria will need teams of doctors and social workers, in particular to be responsible for monitoring patients who are being treated with antiretroviral drugs.

However, even here we see yet another example of how in the original guiding influence of ensuring primary healthcare as a basic human right, as evidenced in the 1980s, the WHO has since retreated to the position of seeing health as a 'commodity' in the context of neoliberal financial globalisation. The WTO is committed to free global trade. As a result of its application to healthcare, free trade has created an increasing health gap in the LDCs.

Just how much is the developed world receiving in this way from the less developed world, which some believe we are aiding? As has been suggested in earlier chapters, it is not a simple matter to assess the costs of training doctors in different economic contexts or to evaluate the impact of the cost on the local economy. However, according to Sen,[13] it is generally assumed that it costs the equivalent of US$ 60,000 to train a GP in the LDCs, and the equivalent of about US$ 12,000 to train a nurse. According to these figures, the LDCs are subsidising developed-world healthcare at a rate of US$ 500 million a year.

African poverty: a familiar story?

When people in the developed world speak of poverty in the LDCs, some of the countries of Africa are never very far from their minds. The very size of Africa means that most major European countries have had colonial connections with it. It is almost as though we spent 300 or so years robbing it of manpower and resources and then suddenly realised that it was poor! In general, there is also a very widespread view that the wealthy world has been pouring aid into Africa for a long time, but that this is proving persistently ineffective because of internal corruption, mismanagement, tribal wars, etc. However, any dispassionate mathematical analysis of Africa brings to light a vastly different story. What few realise is that the outflows of goods, and even of services, from Africa to countries of the developed world far exceed any inflow from the developed world to Africa.

In preparation for the 2005 G8 Summit at Gleneagles in Scotland, the UK Prime Minister, Tony Blair, convened 17 people (including himself) to form a Commission for Africa. He did this because he would be presiding at the Gleneagles talks. Members of this new Commission were invited eclectically on the basis of their individual and personal capacities, rather than openly representing specific governments or nations. Most of the membership is African, and all 17 individuals have varied experience as political leaders, public servants or in the private sector. Their task was also to define the challenges facing Africa and to provide clear recommendations on how to support the changes necessary to reduce poverty in Africa. In their 2004 Report,[14] the Commission emphasised that the African countries must drive their own development and assert control over their own terms of trade.

Promises to Africa at the 2005 G8 Summit

Readers will recall that at the 2005 G8 Summit at Gleneagles, the UK Prime Minister stated that reversing many of the inequities between Africa and the developed world was a matter of importance to him. Having succeeded in extracting a last-minute pledge from Japan, Blair did apparently succeed, and announced that G8 aid to Africa would increase from the current US$ 25 billion to US$ 50 billion by 2010. As we shall see, though, even if that pledge were to be fulfilled, it would still not reverse the excess outflow from Africa.

It is significant, too, that Blair was unable to secure agreement on getting the G8 countries to increase foreign aid to the equivalent of 0.7% of national income by 2015 – and that is *total* foreign aid, not just for Africa. The summit document somewhat obscured this back-pedalling by stating that the EU countries agreed in principle to the derisory 0.7% figure – but it coyly did not mention the USA! Even the tiny 0.7% of the US budget would have made a significant impact, but US President Bush refused to agree to that target. Possibly with tongue in cheek, a number of worthy commentators welcomed this as a G8 breakthrough, especially the US$ 50 billion over the next five years, declaring it to be a major step forward. That meeting ended on an upbeat note with the G8 nations agreeing support for a new deal on trade, cancellation of the debts of the 18 poorest nations and the pledging of universal access to AIDS treatment as needed. The latter was announced almost on the heels of the announcement that the famous 'three by five' target on HIV/AIDS had failed (*see* Chapter 11).

Spokespeople supportive of the G8 intentions could, of course, plead that the G8 deliberations had been sidelined by the terrorist outrages in London on 7 July. Moreover, the Sudan–Darfur events in particular distorted the focus on Africa's other problems. This also gave the UK Prime Minister an opportunity to invoke 'the war on terror' as a reason for deferring real and concrete action on the African poverty issue. As Finfacts Ireland[15] reported Tony Blair as saying:

> All of our achievements for Africa at Gleneagles do not change the
> world tomorrow – it is a beginning, not an end. And none of it today
> will match the same ghastly impact on the cruelty of terror. But it has
> a pride and a hope and humanity at its heart that can lift the shadow
> of terrorism and light the way to a better future.

Brave words indeed, but the rhetoric has had little impact on the problems, as the next section will make clear.

Have we made poverty history?

Following the Gleneagles Summit, there were real expectations that debt reduction deals would be realised. The call of the Commission for Africa and a statement by African Heads of State for a debt compact, including 100% debt forgiveness to the continent, have so far gone unheeded. It will be recalled that the G8 had agreed 10% of the amount needed by more than 60 countries if they were to meet the UN Millennium Development Goal to reduce world poverty by 2015. The Summit had also agreed that Nigeria would benefit by a debt reduction of 60%.

However, within days of the Summit's end it was revealed that the IMF was about to reinterpret these pledges, and several of the G8 countries were requesting that stricter conditions be attached to any debt relief. As we shall see, most of these conditions involve the imposition of onerous reciprocal agreements on the debtor nations to spend aid money through institutions that generate profit for the developed world's stockholders.

Even worse has been the fate of that much-vaunted promise of US$ 50 billion by 2010. Several countries set a timetable for reaching the 0.7% GDP target, but the USA, Canada and Japan have now refused to commit to that target. All in all, many aid agencies have described the impact of the Summit's brave words as rather disappointing. This view was put rather succinctly by Kumi Naidoo, chair of an NGO called 'Global Call to Action against Poverty',[16] when he said of the Gleneagles G8 Summit, and of the noisy street demonstration about it:

> The people have roared, but the G8 have only whispered!

Draining resources out of Africa

In the light of the splendid statements made about African poverty at the G8 Summit in Gleneagles and at the WTO meeting in Hong Kong in 2005, let us reconsider our previous assertion about the extent of the net outflow of resources from that continent. As most readers probably appreciate, the resource drain from Africa began several centuries ago and was consolidated through slavery, colonialism and iniquitous terms of trade. However, it has become much worse over the last four decades through the mediation of the Bretton Woods institutions and the exercise of neoliberal finance in controlling global trade.

Fast-track financial market integration is being promoted across Africa. This trend has been associated with a declining contribution of manufacturing to the GDPs of African nations, accompanied by a rising contribution of credit, real estate, stock-market investment and financial speculation generally. The World Bank itself concedes that Africa now repays more than it receives of outflow in the form of debt repayments equal to those terms of the original loan and, in most African countries, exceeding earnings from exports.[17]

Trade liberalisation under the WTO has exacted about US$ 272 billion since 1986. This has led to dependence on export of primary commodities, and some falling prices for them. African producers find themselves caught in a price trap, as they generate higher production levels that bring in decreasing revenues.

As was stated earlier, Africa is often depicted as a rather unworthy recipient of our aid largesse, but the developed world's exploitation of Africa's non-renewable resources, along with the air and water pollution consequent upon this, have added seriously to Africa's debt burden. The UNDP has estimated that the value of minerals in South African soil fell from US$ 112 billion in 1960 to only US$ 55 billion in 2000! Methods used by the World Bank for measuring resource depletion estimate that a country's potential GDP falls by 9% for every percentage point increase in a country's dependency on extractive resources. Using that formula, we can say that Gabon's people lost US$ 2,241 each in 2000! The negative health impacts of such outflows are obvious, and impinge most heavily on women (and therefore on children), undermining any progress towards the achievement of dignity for the majority of African people.[18]

Neoliberal economists criticise aid programmes to Africa on the grounds that the African countries first need to create a stronger climate for investment and access to markets. Instead, however, in order for African nations to sustain and improve basic welfare programmes, such as making primary healthcare accessible to all, they need to grab back for themselves a percentage of the outflow. One way of doing this would be through Tobin Taxes, as the author suggested in 2000.[19] A Tobin Tax is a small tax on international currency transactions, proposed by James Tobin in 1978 as a means of discouraging short-term capital outflows. Advocates suggested that there should be a tax of 1.025%, and that this money should be used for urgent priorities within the country. The country could also insist on adequate ecological reparation for transnational mining operations.

Between 1990 and 2001, poverty across Africa increased steeply, with 77% of its people surviving on just above US$ 2 a day. As will be seen in Chapter 8, women and children bear the brunt of this burden. African countries fall further behind every day,[20] and as recently as 2005, Christian Aid concluded that:

> Trade liberalisation has cost sub-Saharan Africa US$ 272 billion over the past 20 years. Had they not been forced to liberalise as the price of aid, loans and debt relief, sub-Saharan African countries would have had enough extra income to wipe out their debts and have sufficient left over to pay for every child to be vaccinated and go to school. Two decades of liberalisation has cost sub-Saharan Africa roughly what it has received in aid. Effectively, this aid did no more than compensate African countries for the losses they sustained by meeting the conditions that were attached to the aid they received.[21]

Much of this outflow is, of course, the result of unsustainable rates of compound interest charges on IMF and World Bank debts.

Cost of African debt repayment

As Bond[22] has pointed out, the much-vaunted Gleneagles generosity is based on the assumption that service repayments to lenders in the developed countries are sustainable. However, Africa has already repaid much more than it received in the 1990s because of the compound interest on arrears. In total, Africa repaid

US$ 255 billion – that is, over four times the original 1990 debt. In fact, in some countries, including Cameroon, Gambia, Mauritania, Senegal and Zambia, servicing the debt exceeded the money allocated to healthcare.

Table 6.1 is most instructive in this context.

Table 6.1   Africa's debt and repayments for the period 1980–2000, derived from World Bank Global Finance Tables 2002[23]

Total foreign debt:	US$ 61 billion (1980)	→	US$ 206 billion (2002)
Debt to GDP ratio:	23% (1980)	→	66% (2002)
Loan to repayment ratio:	US$ 9.6 billion: US$ 3.2 billion (1980)	→	US$ 3.2 billion: US$ 9.8 billion (2000)
Net flow:	+US$ 6.4 billion	→	–US$ 6.2 billion
Overall repayment:	US$ 255 billion (1980s–1990s)	*or*	4.02 times original 1980 value

In 1980, with inflow comfortably higher than the debt repayment outflow, Africa continued to pay abnormally high interest to service loans, and did so with new loans. However, by 2000 the net flow deficit was US$ 6.2 billion, so new loans no longer paid the interest on old loans. Those resources were now squeezed from already impoverished economies. For 21 African countries, the debt reached at least 300% of exports by 2002, and for countries such as Sudan, Burundi, Sierra Leone and Guinea-Bissau, it was 15 times greater than annual export earnings.

In at least 16 countries, according to Eric Toussaint, debt inherited from undemocratic governments could be defined as legally 'odious' and therefore eligible for cancellation, since citizens were victimised both in the debt's original accumulation and use of monies against the citizens, and in subsequent demands that it be repaid. These amounts are estimated to exceed 50% of Africa's outstanding debt (*see* Table 6.2).

Table 6.2   Debt repayments for sub-Saharan Africa, 2003, derived from Commission for Africa[24]

	Bilateral lenders ('donor deals')	*Multilateral lenders (World Bank, IMF, African Development Bank)*	*Private lenders*	*Total*
HIPCs (US$ billion)	1.1	1.1	0.1	2.3
Other low-income countries (US$ billion)	1.1	0.7	1.8	3.6
Middle-income countries (US$ billion)	0.3	0.2	2.3	2.7
Total (US$ billion)	2.4	2.0	4.2	8.6

HIPCs, heavily indebted poor countries.

Aid: real and phantom

Many commentators, including this author, have noted that aid to developing nations dropped precipitously after the collapse of the former Soviet Union. The presence of the USSR as a possible competitor for hearts and minds (and resources) in the less developed world kept the USA and the wealthy nations giving. However, once that competition had disappeared, the wealthy west reduced aid substantially. Yet, pre detailed analysis shows that this decline in flow from the developed to the less developed world actually began as far back as the 1960s.

As things stand in 2006, aid from most developed-world countries (the Netherlands, Norway, Denmark and Sweden excepted) is much less than the UN 1970 goal of 0.7%. The USA gives only 0.12% and Japan gives only 0.23%.[25] Action Aid reports that just over a third of the aid sent is 'real', in the sense that it involves people actually receiving money or goods. The rest is 'tied' to projects that involve having to buy parts and/or services from the donor country. Military aid, of course, falls into this category. Levels of aid from developed countries to LDCs are not, on the whole, determined by the real health or other needs of the recipient country, but more often by the strategic or economic needs of the donor country. As I shall be discussing in the final chapter, the only realistic way to ensure that aid from the developed world reaches and benefits the less developed world would be for some agency other than the donor country to determine the amount of aid and what policies should accompany it.

Action Aid's already cited report includes a most illuminating graph (*see* Figure 6.4). The brutal arithmetic is just as damning. In 2003, total aid from the developed world to the less developed world amounted to US$ 69 billion, but of this only US$ 27 billion (less than half!) was 'real' aid. The rest was generating a direct profit for the donor countries.

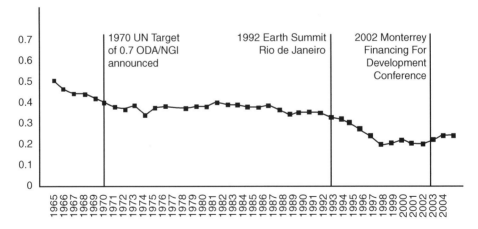

Figure 6.4 Third World aid trends, 1965–2004.

In dealing with this analysis of African poverty and the negative impact of developed-world agencies, I have so far said little about a number of economic and banking issues, such as capital flight (flows in money exchange, etc.), primary commodities export, or even trade in general. Lack of space precludes a more detailed analysis of such economic criteria in this book. However, before bringing this chapter to a close, I would like to touch on the issue of agricultural subsidies, especially in the EU and the USA, and their deleterious impact on the health and other human rights of the LDCs.

How many African people is a French cow worth?

The answer to this question, by the way, is that EU subsidies give each French cow about US$ 2.05 a day. This, as we know, is more than about 70% of African citizens have to live on. I shall leave it to the reader to divide the number of Africans by the number of French cows! What it boils down to is that, in the EU, taxpayers are paying nearly US$ 2.5 billion annually to support the EU dairy industry through the Common Agricultural Policy. As I have already demonstrated with regard to subsidies for US cotton farmers and the impact that these have on cotton farmers in Burkina Faso, the EU 'cow subsidy' effectively ruins the lives of many of the world's already desperately poor people.

Due to overproduction, EU surpluses of milk and milk products are dumped on world markets, using costly export subsidies and thereby undermining farmers in LDCs. The benefits to be gained from this activity – and there are many – go overwhelmingly to the wealthy in the developed world, through profits made by dairy processing, shipping and trading enterprises. It all ties in with the role of transnational corporations (TNCs) and their impact on human rights in the LDCs. Let it be noted, though, with regard to agricultural subsidies, that the NGO Oxfam has taken a strong stand on this issue. It is currently campaigning for an immediate end to EU dairy-export dumping, and for agricultural support to be directed instead to small LDC farmers. That would be an example of 'real' aid!

References

1 World Health Organization. *The World Health Report 1995. Bridging the gaps.* Geneva: World Health Organization; 1995. pp. 12–14.
2 Truman H. *Truman Archives.* Campaign speech, 12 March 1947; www.americanrhetoric.com/speeches/harrytruman (accessed 22 July 2006).
3 Kissinger H. 'Feed the hungry.' Speech at First World Food Conference, 20 April 1974; www.alternet.org (accessed 9 November 2006).
4 Brown G. Speech at Labour Conference in Brighton on 26 September 2005; www.labour.org.uk /news/ac05sb (accessed 24 May 2006).
5 http://geography.about.com/library/weekly/aa071497.htm (accessed 24 May 2006).
6 Nelson-Pallmeyer J. *Brave New World Order.* London: Orbis Publishers; 1992. p. 14.
7 Buchan J, Seccombe I. *Immigration: the need for foreign nurses;* www.migrationwatch.co.uk/ Briefingpapers/health/foreign_nurses (accessed 24 May 2006).
8 Frommel D. 'Global market' in medical workers; www.blythe.org/nytransfer-subs/Africa/Exporting Health (accessed 10 June, 2006).
9 Cessou S. Fruite des cerveaux: l'Afrique part en croisade. *Marchés Tropicaux*, 13 February 2001, p. 12.
10 Mejia A, Pizurki H, Royston E. *Physician and Nurse Migration: analysis and policy immigrations.* Geneva: World Health Organization; 1979. pp. 33–7.
11 UN General Assembly, 23rd Session, Resolution 2417. Outflow of trained professional and technical personnel at all levels from the developing to the developed countries,

its causes, its consequences and practical remedies for the problems resulting from it. 1745th Plenary Session, 17 December 1968.

12 World Health Organization. *Health for All in the Twenty-First Century.* Copenhagen: WHO Regional Office for Europe; 1999. pp. 4–20.

13 Sen A. Health in development. *WHO Bull.* 1999; **77**: 619–23.

14 Commission for Africa. Report, 2004. www.commissionforafrica.org/English/home/newstories.html (accessed 3 June 2006).

15 Finfacts Ireland. 'G8 leaders agree £50 billion African Aid.' www.finfacts.com/irelandbusinessnews/article_10002435.shtml (accessed 3 June 2006).

16 BBC News. 'Government defends G8 aid boost.' Broadcast 5 September 2005; www.news.bbc.co.uk/1/hi/business/4666743.stm (accessed 3 June 2006).

17 Bond P. *The Dispossession of African Wealth at the Cost of African Health.* Regional Network for Equity in Health in East and South-Eastern African (EQUINET), Centre for Economic Justice. EQUINET Discussion Paper No. 30. Harare, Zimbabwe: Training and Research Support Centre; 2006. p. 3.

18 Ibid., p. 8.

19 Macdonald T. *Third World Health Promotion.* Lewiston, NY: Edwin Mellen Press; 2000. p. 106.

20 Bakker I, Gill S. Ontology, method and hypotheses. In: Bakker I, Gill S, editors. *Power, Production and Social Reproduction.* Basingstoke: Palgrave, Macmillan; 2003.

21 Christian Aid. *The Economics of Failure: the real cost of 'free' trade for poor countries.* London: Christian Aid; 2005. p. 2.

22 Bond P, op. cit., p. 8.

23 World Bank. *Global Finance Tables 2002;* www.worldbank.org/annualreport/2002/overview.htm (accessed 4 June 2006).

24 Commission for Africa, op. cit., p. 22.

25 Action Aid. *Real Aid: an agenda for making aid work.* Johannesburg: Action Aid; 2005. p. 2.

Chapter 7

Transnational corporations: instruments for global control

Transnational commerce: robbing the less developed countries

As indicated previously, one of the major impacts of free trade, GATT and GATS has been the penetration into economies of less developed countries (LDCs) by transnational corporations of developed countries. Many of these corporations have entered the country concerned directly as a result of IMF structural adjustment policies. Although such corporations routinely engage in some of the most blatant abuses of human rights (e.g. use of child labour, hazardous working conditions, etc.), it is extraordinarily difficult to establish the details of such abuse or to hold the agencies concerned to account. Neoliberal globalisation has created an ideal climate for such evils. Whatever the rhetoric, the perpetrators are not concerned primarily with human rights, but with creating better dividends for their stockholders.

Increasingly, though, citizens in the developed world are becoming aware of the abuses and are beginning to ask awkward questions. Also, some credit for this must go to the transnational corporations themselves, and in addition the citizens of less developed nations are not remaining passive. They are becoming informed via increasing availability of access to computers, modern methods of communication, etc. The importance of literacy in this respect, as will be discussed in Chapter 10, cannot be overstated. For all these reasons this author is confident that the present scenario will have changes forced upon it.

One of the developed-world-based organisations that is active in this struggle is a group called Global Exchange, which has developed a list of some of the world's worst corporate abusers. It claims that such widely respected corporations as Coca-Cola, Caterpillar, Dow Chemical, Lockheed, Philip Morris, Wal-Mart, Nestlé – and many others – have been complicit in such abuses as assassinations, torture, abduction, environmental degradation, misuse of public funds, violent repression of union activity and other political rights, releasing toxins into the air and water supplies, and even destroying homes. Reinforced by such tactics as exploitation of women, racial discrimination and suborning domestic police and other law and protection agencies, they have created widespread health problems and have weakened many existing methods for remedying these. A number of the companies that have been listed by Global Exchange are currently being sued under the Alien Tort Act. This progressive piece of American legislation makes it possible for citizens of any country to seek redress in US federal courts for violations of international rights and treaties.

At this point it is worthwhile considering precisely what a 'corporation' is and where it stands legally. In the broadest and most general use of the term, a corporation is a business entity that is given many of the same rights as an actual person. That last point is a crucial one, because a corporation is only counted as an individual person with regard to some of their rights, and rarely with regard to their responsibilities. Thus if a worker is killed because inadequate protection or training was given by the corporation that hired him or her, the owner of the corporation cannot be held responsible for the person's death. So, in legal terms, the definition of 'corporation' is changed to make the analogy with a 'person' being 'virtual' or 'fictitious.' Thus the legal definition includes the following phrase: 'corporations exist as virtual or fictitious persons, granting a limited protection to the actual owners of the corporation.'[1] This limitation of liability is one of the principal advantages of incorporation. It constitutes a major incentive for smaller businesses to become corporations, especially if they are involved in particularly hazardous projects or in ones that are highly litigated.

In general, trade union organisation is so strong in the developed world that adherence to health and safety legislation protects workers from the more blatant abuses of corporate power, although this is by no means always the case. However, in the less developed world, such protection is usually minimal or even absent. One could write several books about the details, but we shall content ourselves with a brief description of each of the 14 major offenders listed by the Global Exchange. Some of them are household words in modern society. However, one should not get the impression that the situations mentioned are uniquely bad. Even the horrendous Bhopal disaster (Dow Chemical Company – Union Carbide) is more remarkable for the spectacularly large number of people killed in one place than for the level of cavalier exploitation behind it.

First, however, we shall consider what international instrumentalities pronounce specifically on the human rights associated with health and safety in the workplace or other human rights associated with employment.

In articles 23 to 25 of the Universal Declaration of Human Rights, labour rights are outlined, clearly stating the universal right to just and favourable conditions in the workplace, equal pay for equal work, unions, reasonable working hours, and 'a standard of living adequate for health and well-being.' Transnational corporations (TNCs), as workplaces, have a responsibility to uphold these rights and to exert discipline within their structure when these rights are not respected.[2]

The people of the world would have much less to protest if the TNCs upheld their responsibilities with regard to labour rights and all human rights, but this is not the case. The International Tribunal on Workers' Human Rights in 1997 found that articles 3, 4, 8, 12–14, 19, 20 and 22–25 of the Universal Declaration of Human Rights were being violated under the current global economic system of laissez-faire capitalism.[3]

In what could be called more indirect violations of human rights, but with consequences that are just as serious, TNCs aid and abet the continual destruction of the environment, the displacement of indigenous peoples, the theft of common intellectual property, and economic dependence. This economic dependence is part of a cycle that goes beyond the dependence of workers on TNCs to earn a living in areas of high unemployment, while at the same time making it far more hazardous for them to do so.

With the support of global power structures such as the World Bank and the International Monetary Fund (IMF), TNCs drain countries of their resources, take advantage of lax laws in poorer nations, and maintain the economic power of the developed world. The World Bank and the IMF use the promise of loans to initiate economic changes in the LDCs, while the TNCs take advantage of these changes and send the profits back to the developed-world countries. The LDCs remain economically dependent on the developed countries, with the violation of fundamental human rights as a main support beam within the global economic power structure.

To be an informed activist, or even just to be informed, it helps to understand the concrete human rights violations that result from the globalised economic power structure that is in place today. Since transnational corporations are major players in this structure, this chapter will delineate some of the direct and indirect human rights violations for which they are responsible.

Dow Chemical Company and the Bhopal disaster

Dow Chemical Company is a large US-owned firm, and Union Carbide Corporation (UCC) is one of its offshoots in the USA. One of UCC's affiliates in India is Union Carbide Limited (UCIL). In fact, at the time of the disaster, UCC owned just over 50% of the equity of UCIL. In addition, it maintained extensive corporate, managerial, technical and operational control over UCIL.

During the night of 2 December 1984, a huge amount (around 36 tons) of toxic gases leaked from a pesticide plant in Bhopal, the capital city of Madhya Pradesh State in Central India. The main component of the leaked gas was no less than 24 tons of methyl isocyanate (MIC), together with other lethal toxins such as hydrogen cyanide itself, nitrous oxide and carbon monoxide. Over the next 72 hours around 7,200 people died horribly. Many more (probably 20,000 or more) were incapacitated either by gas inhalation, leading to blindness, neurological damage and impaired respiration, or by physical injuries such as broken limbs, crushing injuries, etc., sustained during the stampede to escape. During the ensuing 22 years, in excess of 100,000 people have been left with chronic illnesses that prevent them from working.

Survivors, and those representing them, have been assiduous in trying to use the US courts, and those in India itself, to gain recognition of such a gross violation of their human rights, but so far they have been unsuccessful. The only redress – a derisory 'goodwill' financial settlement between Dow Chemical Company and the Indian Government – has so far failed to trickle down to the actual victims. However, legal responsibility has been avoided. UCC has consistently argued that the Bhopal plant was not under either its management or its control, despite its corporate, managerial, technical and operational control over UCIL, as mentioned above. Dow try to claim that UCIL themselves are completely responsible. Dow Chemicals, which took over UCC in 2001, 17 years after the event, has made a public statement that they have absolutely no responsibility, either for the leak itself or for its subsequent impact on health. They also deny any responsibility for the broader environmental pollution caused by the plant. As for the UCC, it has refused to appear before any court in India. Finally, the Supreme Court of India endorsed a final settlement that has left survivors living in penury.[4]

The pause that refreshes: Coca-Cola

Coca-Cola is so popular as a pleasant, sparkling and stimulating drink worldwide that it is difficult to associate it with serious human rights abuses. Think again! Of course, one could write a great deal about how bad Coca-Cola is for one's health, but on the larger scale of the deleterious effects of the Coca-Cola Corporation on health, we are not primarily concerned in this account with its physiological impact as a food supplement! The Coca-Cola Corporation produces not only the familiar fizzy dark brown beverage, but also a variety of other fizzy drinks and even fizzy water. In the process of carrying out these activities, especially in LDCs, it massively violates human rights and environmental sustainability.

When we speak of Coca-Cola, we are speaking of a multimillion-dollar global enterprise. In Colombia, since April 2003 a group that calls itself the campaign to 'Stop Killer Coke' has been active. It started at a particular Coca-Cola bottling plant in Colombia, but is widely supported financially by US human rights groups, and is now active in a number of LDCs as well as in the developed world. Stop Killer Coke involvement in Colombia came about when it supported a trade union, Sinaltrainal, whose membership was drawn largely from the food and drink industry. Managers of Coca-Cola bottling plants in Colombia are currently facing trial for having paid paramilitary death squads to assassinate eight Sinaltrainal activists. They are also accused of several accounts of kidnapping and torture, as well as the falsification of evidence leading to trade unionists being arrested for charges of terrorism. These cases have been ongoing since 31 March 2003, when a US district court ruled that cases of human rights violations by paramilitaries on behalf of Coca-Cola, brought by Sinaltrainal, could proceed. This was an example of the application of the Aliens Tort Claims Act (ACTA), discussed previously.[5]

Coca-Cola has also been implicated in various violations of environmental protection laws in Colombia, Turkey, India and elsewhere. In Kerala State in India the Coca-Cola plant at Plachimada was found to have released cadmium, a known carcinogen, as a waste product. They got rid of it by selling the material to local farmers as a fertiliser, without advising them of the cancer risk involved in handling the product. The 'fertiliser' soon found its way into local wells. The BBC TV programme, *Face the Facts*,[6] took samples from some of the wells and had the water analysed at the University of Exeter. There it was not only established that cadmium-rich waste was useless as a fertiliser, but also that the waste product contained lead, another toxic metal, in addition to cadmium. The BBC tests established that the levels of these toxic metals were 'well above those set by the World Health Organization.'

The same BBC programme also stated that the local community interests were taking the Coca-Cola plant to court because of its prodigious exploitation of local groundwater, claiming that this could incur drought and other serious ecological damage. Local politicians claimed that this disruption of water supplies was compromising not only access to drinking water, but also the irrigation of rice paddies.

Coca-Cola breached Indian law at its Plachimada bottling plant in southern India by continuing its 'trial operations' on 8 August 2005. The Kerala State Pollution Control Board subsequently ordered Coke to 'stop production of all kinds of products with immediate effect' at the plant on 19 August. The Plachimada plant was originally pressured to stop operations in March 2004, due to complaints from the local community about pollution and an alarming loss of potable water.

According to the India Resource Centre, Coca-Cola's operations have resulted in extreme water shortages, as well as the contamination of soil and groundwater. Coca-Cola has effectively avoided responding to the Indian government, and others, on the issue of water contamination due to cadmium in the Plachimada plant's sludge. Two previous orders by the Kerala Pollution Control Board were ignored. One of these orders called for Coca-Cola to build an effluent treatment facility to deal with waste water, while the other required the company to pipe potable water into communities to meet the needs of residents most vulnerable to water shortages.[7]

The Indian Resource Centre also notes that Coca-Cola was implicated in a bribery scandal involving a member of the Kerala Pollution Control Board, namely KV Indulal. In 2003, Mr Indulal maintained that the level of pollution coming from Coca-Cola's bottling plant in Plachimada met acceptable standards. Shortly thereafter, the BBC and the Kerala Pollution Control Board launched separate investigations, both of which found grim environmental conditions that exceeded tolerable levels.

The dossier on Coca-Cola is large, involving similar violations of the health and safety of workers and populations affected by bottling and manufacturing plants in Turkey, Indonesia, Panama, a number of African countries and even in the USA itself (on several occasions). I shall close this brief account with a quote from *Multinational Monitor*.[8]

> Coca-Cola was named as one of the 'worst corporations of 2004' by the *Multinational Monitor*. The company was added to the list for the 'extensive documentation of rampant violence committed against Coke's unionised workforce by paramilitary forces.' The publication cites an April 2004 report from a delegation headed by New York City Council Member Hiram Monserrate that says, 'To date, there have been a total of 179 major human rights violations of Coca-Cola's workers, including nine murders. Family members of union activists have been abducted and tortured. Union members have been fired for attending meetings. ... Most troubling to the delegation were the persistent allegations that paramilitary violence against workers was carried out with the knowledge of and likely under the direction of the company managers. ... Shockingly, company officials admitted to the delegation that they had never investigated the ties between plant managers and paramilitaries.'

Caterpillar in Palestine

Caterpillar is the only corporation listed by Global Exchange whose human rights activities seem to have been largely geographically constrained, in this case to the Palestinian–Israeli theatre of conflict. A clear account of the situation is given by Nick Dearden and Joe Zacune.[9] Nick Dearden is Senior Campaign Officer for the anti-poverty charity, War on Want (www.waronwant.org). Joseph Zacune is a campaigner and researcher on issues linked to corporations and the arms trade. In the context of the Palestinian–Israeli conflict, we are accustomed to reading accounts of Palestinians firing homemade mortar bombs into Israeli territory and using suicide bombers to penetrate Israel in person. Likewise, we read of how

Israel responds, by using the most modern military hardware and a well-equipped air force against Palestinian positions.

However, in terms of routine human rights violations, Israel's most potent weapon seems to be a particular type of Caterpillar bulldozer. Dearden and Zacune quote the UN Special Rapporteur on the right to food as saying: 'Caterpillar's D9 bulldozers have been responsible for destroying agricultural farms, greenhouses, ancient olive groves ... numerous Palestinian homes and sometimes human lives.'

The last-mentioned item is rather understated, as the number of lives lost as a result of the use of D9s has actually been enormous. Since 2002, the Israeli army has used these machines to flatten over 4,000 homes, thereby rendering nearly 100,000 Palestinians homeless, killing some who were unable to get out in time, injuring thousands and traumatising many more. For instance, the effect on young children requires little imagination. These demolitions, according to Israeli apologists, are carried out as 'punishment' on the people of areas that are believed to be harbouring terrorists. If this is so, it is clearly illegal under international law. Even worse, Israel's own human rights organisation, B'Tselem, found that in half the cases there was no evidence linking the targeted buildings or their occupants to acts against Israel!

Palestinians are currently experiencing poverty levels comparable with those in some of the poorest parts of sub-Saharan Africa. The UN reports that Palestine bears the 'effects of a terrible natural disaster, though one created by people and politics.' A key cause of this poverty is the destruction of agricultural land, the only possible source of livelihood open to many Palestinians. Caterpillar bulldozers have been used to tear up extensive areas of cultivated land, destroying thousands of olive groves and citrus trees. The destruction of wells, storage tanks and water pumps has severely limited access to drinking water.

In Jenin camp, which is home to 14,000 refugees, Caterpillar's D9 bulldozers were a key component of Operation Defensive Shield, the 'most extensive and severe' human rights violation since 1967 (B'Tselem). The Hawashin district of the camp was levelled and many residents were given no advance notice of this. Many were buried alive, including paraplegic Jamal Suliman. According to his mother, 'the bulldozer wouldn't wait even one minute so that we could take Jamal out of the house.'

During a raid on a refugee camp in Rafah in May 2004, UN Special Rapporteur on human rights John Dugard noted that 'Homes have been destroyed in a purely purposeless manner. Bulldozers have savagely dug up roads, including electricity, sewerage and water lines, in a brutal display of power.' A total of 298 homes were destroyed in Rafah in a single month.

Perhaps, however, the bulldozers are best described by the experiences of two young people on either side of the Occupation. Israeli Army D9 operator Moshe Nissim describes his experience of Jenin: 'I had no mercy for anybody. I would erase anyone with the D9. When I was told to demolish a house, I took the opportunity to bring down some more houses.' His unit was commended for outstanding service. On the other side was 23-year-old US peace activist Rachel Corrie. At an International Solidarity Movement demonstration, she stood in front of a Palestinian home, trying to prevent its demolition. The D9 driver initially dumped sand on her, and later drove over her as demolition proceeded. Rachel died of her injuries.

Terrible as all of this is, many readers may well wonder how the manufacturers of the D9 can be held accountable for the use of its machines for human rights abuses. The CEO of Caterpillar, James Owens, was not after all personally driving the vehicles that committed the outrages. However, a group of concerned Caterpillar shareholders in the USA raised the matter with him in a resolution in 2004 that asked whether 'Caterpillar's directors can reconcile acquiescence with the use of the D9s by Israel with the company's Code of Worldwide Business Conduct.'

Such is the legal status of corporations that it appears that the answer to that rhetorical question is 'Yes.' One of Caterpillar's slogans is that 'We do well by doing well around the world.' In fact, another comment from Caterpillar's Worldwide Business Code is 'We believe that our success should also contribute to the quality of life and the prosperity of communities.'

Dearden and Zacune go on to report that, when UN Special Rapporteur Jean Ziegler wrote to James Owens in May 2004, expressing concern that Caterpillar may be violating the right of Palestinians to food, guaranteed by the International Covenant on Economic, Social and Cultural Rights, he received no reply!

The complicity of Caterpillar in such violations of human rights is further underlined by the fact that they advertise D9 bulldozers in various conflict zones, such as Iraq and Afghanistan. Furthermore, many of the D9s that are purchased from Caterpillar for use in Israel's Palestinian incursions are paid for by US taxpayers.

In June 2005, the ethics of Caterpillar's activities in the Middle East hit the headlines in the UK because of the involvement of the Church of England.[10] At the Nottingham meeting of the latter on 21 June 2005, the following resolution was passed unanimously by the Anglican Consultative Council.

> The Anglican Consultative Council:
>
> a) welcomes the September 22nd 2004 statement by the Anglican Peace and Justice Network on the Israeli/Palestine Conflict (pages 12–14 of the Report)
>
> b) commends the resolve of the Episcopal Church (USA) to take appropriate action where it finds that its corporate investments support the occupation of Palestinian lands or violence against innocent Israelis, and
>
> i) commends such a process to other Provinces having such investments, to be considered in line with their adopted ethical investment strategies
>
> ii) encourages investment strategies that support the infrastructure of a future Palestine State
>
> c) requests of the Office of the Anglican Observer to the United Nations, through or in association with the UN Working Committee on Peace in the Middle East, as well as through this Council, and as a priority of that Office, to support and advocate the implementation of UN Resolutions 242 and 338 directed towards peace, justice and co-existence in the Holy Land.

Naturally this caused considerable controversy in church circles. The more evangelical wing opposed the Consultative Council statement as 'anti-Semitic', but the debate has served to bring the whole issue to the attention of a far wider swathe of the British public and the media than would otherwise have been the case.

How Wal-Mart is remaking our world

The trade name 'Wal-Mart', rather like that of Coca-Cola, tends to have a fairly innocent reputation in the eyes of many, linked as it is with its employees being called 'associates' and its determination to strip frills so as to offer goods at the lowest possible price to consumers. However, its impact in the less developed world, and even in its country of origin, the USA, has been such as to prevent access by its employees to primary healthcare and to remove even further the realisation of any global mandate of basic human rights.

Wal-Mart is the largest TNC in the world, owning in excess of 5,000 stores and employing nearly two million workers worldwide. It makes it into the list of the 14 most egregious corporations in violating human rights because of such practices as enforced overtime, sex discrimination, and illegal use of child labour and aggressive union-busting. It fails to provide health insurance for over half its staff. It is its low price policy that lies at the root of all of these abuses and its disastrous impact on health and other rights in the less developed world.

Wal-Mart maintains its low prices in two ways – by unrelenting exploitation of labour, especially overseas, and by forcing its suppliers to compete with one another to produce goods at the lowest possible wholesale prices. Health and safety law, and effective trade unions, cushion most of the developed-world Wal-Mart employees from most (but not all) of these abuses, but have dramatically lowered standards of life in its overseas plants – including those of its suppliers.

Lawsuits against Wal-Mart have been filed on behalf of its suppliers, including sweatshops in China, Indonesia, Bangladesh and Swaziland. As well as workers in their workplaces being denied even the low minimum wages mandated in those countries, they are routinely expected to work overtime without compensation, on top of a regular seven-day working week, and they are denied legally required healthcare. In addition, such violations as locked washrooms/toilets, compulsory pregnancy tests and instant dismissal for complaints or any attempt to join unions are common.[11]

Of the 10 richest people in the world, five are from the family that owns Wal-Mart. In fact, despite its claim to slash profits in pursuit of the lowest possible prices for consumers, it clears profits of about US$ 7 billion a year, making it one of the most profitable corporations on earth. S Robson Wotton, the chief owner of Wal-Mart, was ranked in London's 'Rich List' in 2001 as the wealthiest person in the world. He had declared a personal fortune of US$ 65 billion, and thus topped Bill Gates as first in that league.[12]

Chevron: polluter extraordinaire

Chevron is a huge multinational petrochemical company, and has been declared guilty of some of the worst environmental and human rights abuses in the world.[13] One of its predecessors was Texaco (which was subsidised by Chevron in

2001) during the years 1968–1992, which was responsible for incalculable human rights violations in Ecuador. In effect, it created what became known as a 'Rainforest Chernobyl' in that country by leaving in excess of 600 unlined pits in Ecuador's rainforest and dumping 18 billion gallons of toxic production water into rivers used for bathing, fishing and supplies of drinking water. As a consequence, the local people suffered a catalogue of health problems, including cancers, skin lesions, blindness, birth defects and spontaneous abortions.

In Nigeria, Chevron has violently repressed locally organised peaceful opposition to oil extraction. It even hired private military personnel to open fire on the protesters. In this, it was also involved with Shell (which is not listed among the 14 worst corporations) in local resistance in the Ogoni region.[14]

Chevron has even significantly offended in violating the health rights of US workers. One of its largest domestic refineries is in Richmond, California, and it processes around 350,000 barrels of oil a day. Consequently, local residents suffer from a range of serious health problems, including lupus, skin irritations, liver and kidney problems, cancer, and cardiac and visual problems.

However, Chevron behaved even more outrageously overseas. In 2004, 15 Burmese (Myanmarese) villages accused a Chevron subsidiary, the Unocal Corporation, of a range of human rights abuses, including rape, summary executions, torture, forced labour and forced migration.

Dyn Corp: security against human rights

Because of the capacity of TNCs for practising exploitation in the less developed world, under the present favourable climate created for this by the Bretton Woods institutions, it should come as no surprise that the fastest growing sector of the global economy is the provision of private security firms to protect TNCs from the people they are exploiting! It is now an industry valued at US$ 100 billion annually,[15] and it is virtually an unregulated industry. Dyn Corp is one such corporation, even going so far as to provide mercenary forces and not merely security men, and amply demonstrating the industry's potential for abusing human rights.

Its range on contracted activities would do credit to any army invading several countries, as it fields security forces in Afghanistan and African oil fields, trains Iraqi police forces under contract to the US government, and eradicates cocaine production units in Colombia. It has even been involved in protecting business premises in post-hurricane New Orleans. The product of Dyn Corp consists of trained corps of 'hired guns', and they are not constrained by legal niceties such as human rights. For instance, as part of its contract to eradicate cocaine production in Colombia, thousands of Ecuadorean peasant farmers (the two countries share a border) suffered a number of adverse health effects, because the herbicide that Dyn Corp used was highly toxic. Corp Watch has reported similar scenarios from various countries.

Attendant upon such 'unregulated' use of overriding force, it would not be surprising to find other, non-industrial human rights violations being practised. In Bosnia, in March 2001, a mechanic employed by Dyn Corp blew the whistle on the fact that their employers engaged in rape and in trading girls as young as 12 years as sex slaves. Corp Watch quotes from the lawsuit filed by the mechanic concerned: 'Employees and supervisors engaged in perverse, illegal and inhumane behaviour and were purchasing illegal weapons, women and forged passports.'[16] The response of Dyn Corp was to dismiss the whistleblower and then to transfer all of the accused employees to other countries! Eventually some of these employees were dismissed, but no one has ever been prosecuted.

KBR (Kellogg, Brown and Root): Halliburton Corporation

The Halliburton Corporation is probably best known to most readers because of its involvement in profitable activities in the prosecution of the Iraqi war, and its various links with the White House. Much of its popular notoriety arises from its imaginative approaches to accountancy and book-keeping, but its major business activity is the provision of support services for the US military.

The systematic violation of human rights became apparent gradually between 2001 and 2003, when auditors on US defence panels began to look into some bizarre examples of overcharging for imported gasoline. In June 2005, a previously confidential audit, ordered by the Pentagon, questioned expenditures of US\$ 1.4 billion. In 2002 the company had paid US\$ 2 million to settle a US Justice Department lawsuit that accused KBR of inflating contract prices for petrol supplies to Fort Ord (Army) Base in California.

The impact of the Halliburton Corporation on the less developed world is due principally to their hiring of huge contract armies of labour from Pakistan, Afghanistan and elsewhere to work at US-sponsored reconstruction projects in Iraq. These civilian workers have thereby become part of the largest civilian workforce ever hired in support of a US invasion. The human rights problems have arisen thick and fast, with regard both to workers themselves and to Iraqi civilians. Once the civilian workers have left their own countries and ended up in Iraq, their legal status becomes problematic. They are treated in ways that violate health and safety standards almost anywhere else in the world. They are routinely worked in excess of International Labour Organization (ILO) rules, 10 or more hours a day, 7 days a week. Lack of adequate medical care or even minimal provision for such care is common. In their dealings with the civilian population of Iraq, these workers themselves commit large numbers of human rights abuses, many of which cannot be traced accurately.

Monsanto Chemicals

This corporation has been discussed by the author in a previous publication.[17] It is by far the largest marketer of genetically modified seeds in the world, dominating somewhere between 70% and 100% of the market for such crops as soy, cotton, wheat and corn. It is most noted for its product 'Round-Up', which is sold as a pesticide. 'Round-Up' is largely composed of glyphosate, and it has been shown that although it is effective if used in limited quantities over a short time, it is ultimately a toxin that has a cumulative effect on the soil. Plants on which it is used gradually become infertile over two or three growing seasons, and this compels farmers to purchase genetically modified Round-Up Ready Seed, which is resistant to the herbicide.

Obviously, this brings in its train a cycle of dependency on both the weedkiller itself and the seed that is resistant to it. Both of the products are patented and protected by TRIPS, and Monsanto alone can determine the price for them. An added dimension of this economic violation of human rights is the fact that the pesticide is documented to be carcinogenic, and to cause skin disorders, spontaneous abortions, premature births and damage to the nervous system and the lining of the gastrointestinal tract.

As if these abuses were not enough, the India Committee of the Netherlands and the International Labour Rights Fund have accused Monsanto of employing child labour. It is estimated that, in India, 12,375 children work in cottonseed production for farmers paid by Monsanto, and in various Indian and multi-national seed companies.

Pfizer: from Viagra to AIDS

The exact basis on which Pfizer, one of several large pharmaceutical TNCs, should have been selected as one of the 'worst 14' corporations by Corp Watch is not entirely clear, but its role as a manufacturer and distributor of HIV/AIDS treatments brings its practices into sharp conflict with basic health rights in the poorer countries. It is also the largest pharmaceutical company in the world.

In addition to Viagra, Zoloft, Zithromax and Norvasc, Pfizer produces the drug fluconazole (an antifungal used by AIDS patients, among others) under the name of Diflucan, and sells it at inflated prices that most poor people cannot afford. The company refuses to grant generic licences for fluconazole to governments in countries such as Brazil, South Africa and the Dominican Republic, where patients are forced to pay $20 per weekly pill, although the average national wage is only $120 per month.

Pfizer also values shareholder profits over safety standards. In Europe in 2005, it withdrew from scientific studies of a new class of AIDS drugs called CCR5 inhibitors, choosing instead to rush its own untested CCR5 inhibitor on to the European market without full information about the drug's side-effects.[18]

Much more will be said about the marketing of antiretroviral drugs and other activities of pharmaceutical TNCs with regard to the violation of basic human rights in Chapter 11 on the growing HIV/AIDS pandemic and its consequences.

Suez-Lyonnais Des Eaux

The many issues arising from the lack of equity with regard to access to safe water have been dealt with in Chapter 4. Suffice it to say here that Suez-Lyonnais is regarded by Corp Watch[19] as the 'worst perpetrator of abuses arising from the privatisation of water.' This French company's profit of billions of US dollars comes directly from the violation of the human rights of poor people living in the less developed world, where thousands lack access to potable water. In addition, they are now faced with rapidly rising prices for privatised water.

To quote Corp Watch directly:

> Suez goes by many names around the world – Onedeo, SITA and others – to mask its worldwide net of controversial activities. In Manila, Philippines, after seven years of water privatisation under a Suez company (Maynilad Water) contract, studies showed that water rates increased in some neighbourhoods by 400 to 700 per cent. These studies also showed that the negligence of the company

resulted in cholera and gastroenteritis outbreaks that killed six people and severely sickened 725 people in Manila's Tondo district.

In Bolivia, a Suez company (Agues de Illiman) left 200,000 people without access to water, and caused a revolt when it tried to charge between £335 and £445 to connect a private home to the water supply. Countless people were unable to afford such charges in a country whose yearly per capita GDP is £915.

Unfortunately, the IMF and World Bank are playing a key role in pushing water privatisation all over the world. Many countries have been required to open up their water supply to private companies as a condition for receiving IMF loans, and the World Bank has approved millions of dollars in loans for the privatisation of water systems.

Lockheed Martin and your health!

Lockheed Martin at least does not claim that its products are intended to be health related, as it is the world's largest military contractor! Its violations of basic human rights, such as the right to health, stem almost exclusively from the fact that it has made enormous profits through the use of its products by developed-world powers in pursuing their interests in LDCs. As Corp Watch rather succinctly states, 'Providing satellites, planes, missiles and other high-tech items to the Pentagon has kept the profits rolling in. Since President George W Bush's election in 2000, the company's stock value has tripled.'[20]

The Centre for Corporate Policy, which is an active NGO in the USA, and one highly critical of the war in Iraq, observes that Lockheed was linked from the beginning with the prosecution of the war.[21] They claim that Lockheed's Vice President, Bruce Jackson, helped to draft the US Republican Party's foreign policy platform in 2000. It is surely no coincidence that he was a key player in the so-called 'Project for a New America Century', which is generally perceived as having been the intellectual incubator of the Iraq war. It clearly illustrates the point that the aims of neoliberal economics coincide with those of global control of finance by US and other developed-world corporations, and that the military of those governments are but instruments in the realisation of these aims.

Corp Watch goes on to observe that:

> Lockheed Martin is not the only defence contractor that goes behind the scenes to influence public policy, but it is one of the worst. Stephen J Hadley, who now has Condoleeza Rice's old job as Assistant to the President for National Security Affairs, was formerly a partner in a DC law firm representing Lockheed Martin. He is only one of the beneficiaries of the so-called revolving door between the military industries and the 'civilian' national security apparatus. These war profiteers have a profound and illegitimate influence on our country's international policy decisions.[22]

The Ford Motor Company, Nestlé and Philip Morris

The last three of the '14' worst corporate offenders are the Ford Motor Company, Nestlé and Philip Morris. The author has written extensively on the activities of the last two,[23,24] and would suggest that the reader consults these references for a more detailed account. With regard to Ford, again the author is not entirely sure how it was decided which corporations were the 14 worst ones with regard to human rights violations. Most of the case against Ford focuses on its grossly negative impact on environmental sustainability with regard to carbon emissions which, even though it is taking place largely in the USA, has a global impact. These environmental issues will be dealt with in Chapter 14.

Every year since 1999, the US Environmental Protection Agency (EPA) has ranked Ford vehicles of all types as having the worst overall fuel economy[25] of any US-manufactured automobile. In fact, it pointed out that Ford's 2006 car and track fleet has a lower average fuel efficiency than did Henry Ford's original Model T. The Ford Corporation is also at the bottom of this league when it comes to controlling greenhouse gas emissions. The US-based Union of Concerned Scientists is quoted as saying that 'Ford has the absolute worst heat-trapping gas (petrol) emissions performance of all the major US automobiles.' According to Ford's own sustainability report, between 2003 and 2004 the company's US fleet-wide fuel economy decreased, while its carbon dioxide emissions increased.

In addition, Ford has lobbied actively against the efforts of legislators to increase fuel economy standards.[26]

More about Nestlé and Philip Morris

Since the author's last published commentaries on these firms, enough new information has come to light to suggest that both of them continue to violate human rights and try to avoid complying with the legislation in various countries that is designed to curb this excess. To quote directly from Corp Watch:[27]

> The problem of illegal and forced child labour is rampant in the chocolate industry, because more than 40% of the world's cocoa supply comes from the Ivory Coast, a country that the US State Department estimates had approximately 10,900 child labourers working in hazardous conditions on cocoa farms. In 2001, Save the Children Canada reported that 15,000 children between 9 and 12 years old, many from impoverished Mali, had been tricked or sold into slavery on West African cocoa farms, many for just $30 each.
>
> Nestlé, the third largest buyer of cocoa from the Ivory Coast, is well aware of the tragically unjust labour practices taking place on the farms, with which it continues to do business. Nestlé and other chocolate manufacturers agreed to end the use of abusive and forced child labour on cocoa farms by July 1, 2005, but they failed to do so.
>
> Nestlé is also notorious for its aggressive marketing of infant formula in poor countries in the 1980s. Because of this practice, Nestlé is still one of the most boycotted corporations in the world, and its infant formula is still controversial. In Italy in 2005, police seized more than two million litres of Nestlé infant formula that was contaminated with the chemical isopropylthioxanthone (ITX).

Additionally, violations of labour rights are reported from Nestlé factories in numerous countries. In Colombia, Nestlé replaced the entire factory staff with lower-wage workers and did not renew their collective employment contract.[28]

As for Philip Morris, that firm's name has changed to Altria. It is still the world's largest cigarette corporation, as well as the most profitable one. As the author has pointed out previously,[29] it has shifted strongly into markets in the LDCs in response to increasing concern about tobacco use in developed countries. The World Health Organization predicts that global deaths due to smoking-related illnesses will nearly double (compared with 2004 levels) by 2020, but that more than 75% of these deaths will be in the LDCs.[30]

References

1 Wise Geek. *What is a Corporation?*; www.wisegeek.com/what-is-a-corporation.htm (accessed 22 June 2006).
2 Universal Declaration of Human Rights: Regional Information Centre for Western Europe. www.un.org/rights/HRToday/declar.htm (accessed 22 June 2006).
3 Whitenton C. *Trans-National Corporations and the Violation of Human Rights. Introduction.* Georgia Institute of Technology, 19 February 2005; http://human rights,gatech.edu/tnchr1/php (accessed 22 June 2006).
4 Wikipedia Encyclopaedia. *Bhopal Disaster;* http://en.wikipedia.org/wiki/Bhopal_Disaster (accessed 22 June 2006).
5 *Morning Star,* 20 May 2003, p. 7.
6 *BBC News,* 24 July 2003.
7 India Resource Centre; www.indiaresource.org/news/2005/2001.html (accessed 22 June 2006).
8 Ethics of Coca-Cola. *Multinational Monitor,* 1 December 2004; www.coopamerica.org/programs/rs/profile.cfm?id=204 (accessed 22 June 2006).
9 Dearden N, Zacune J. Caterpillar: making a killing in Palestine?; http://zmagazine.zmag.org./May 2005/dearden0505.html (accessed 22 June 2006).
10 Text from Anglican Communion websites. www.catdestroyshomes.org/article.php?list=class8class=3 (accessed 12 November 2006).
11 Corp Watch. The 14 Worst Corporate Offenders. www.corpwatch.org/article.php?id=12869 (accessed 22 June 2006).
12 Beyond McDonald's 'Comprehensive anti-War Mart info digest'; www.mcspotlight.org/beyond/companies/antiwalmart.htm (accessed 22 June 2006).
13 Corp Watch, op. cit., p. 2.
14 MacDonald T. *Health, Trade and Human Rights.* Oxford: Radcliffe Publishing; 2006. p. 11.
15 Corp Watch, op. cit., p. 5.
16 Corp Watch, op. cit., p. 10.
17 Macdonald T, op. cit., p. 8.
18 Corp Watch, op. cit., p. 4.
19 Corp Watch, op. cit., p. 6.
20 Corp Watch, op. cit., p. 3.
21 Centre for Corporate Policy; www.corporatepolicy.org (accessed 22 June 2006).
22 Corp Watch, op. cit., p. 3.
23 MacDonald T. *Third World Health: hostage to First World wealth.* Oxford: Radcliffe Publishing; 2005. pp.117–61.
24 MacDonald T. *Health, Trade and Human Rights.* Oxford: Radcliffe Publishing; 2006. pp. 61–81.

25 Ibid., p. 3.
26 Corp Watch, op. cit., p. 5.
27 Corp Watch, op. cit., p. 5.
28 Corp Watch, op. cit., p. 6.
29 MacDonald T. *Third World Health: hostage to First World wealth.* Oxford: Radcliffe Publishing; 2005. p. 136.
30 World Health Organization. 'Smoking will kill more people in the developing countries'; www.reason.com/0201/fe.bd.who.shtml (accessed 22 June 2006).

Chapter 8

Gender equality as a basic right to health

Disempowered women and disempowered communities

Compared with men, women are disempowered all over the world. However, their levels of disempowerment are far greater in the less developed countries (LDCs) than in the developed countries, and in terms of their disempowerment as a consequence of neoliberal approaches to financial control there is no sisterhood to speak of. Even while being relatively disadvantaged by comparison with their male colleagues, First World women (as much as men) control the levers that so hideously disempower women in LDCs. In terms of the UN Charter's aim of global human rights, the issue of gender equality is far from being academic. Disempowerment of women itself disempowers much more than 50% of the human race. It is largely women who, at the ground level, make decisions about how to allocate food and other resources for children, and to the extent that women are disempowered, entire families and communities are also disempowered.

We have made huge progress in these matters in the developed world, even though we still have a long way to go. Globally speaking, however, despite numerous international agreements affirming their human rights, women remain much more likely than men to be poor, malnourished and illiterate. As we shall see, these three attributes are intimately linked, and illiteracy in particular is virtually a guarantee of disempowerment (*see* Chapter 10). Disempowerment tends to replicate itself. Once a woman begins life as culturally, socially and even institutionally disempowered, she usually ends up with less access than her brothers to medical care, property ownership, exercise of choice in developing and applying her talents socially, further training and, of course, empowerment. Women become increasingly vulnerable to the routine of domestic violence and much less likely to be politically active.

Of enormous importance both to community welfare and to personal fulfilment is the degree of control that a woman has in controlling her own fertility. This has to be recognised as a bedrock human right if we are to make any significant progress toward the millennium goals. The ability to plan one's family in terms of how it is to be nurtured requires ongoing access to education, for instance, so that constraints placed on women by culture, traditions, religion or law quickly impact on the wider community. To do this properly, a woman must have access to healthcare – both for herself and for her family. Likewise, her voice has to be heard in political decision making at all levels.

Issues to be addressed: targets to be met

Broadly speaking, low status among women is associated with large family size, and this of course is linked to poverty. Enhancement of a population's status is likewise associated with easily accessible reproductive and health programmes. Scientific opinion now suggests that the roles that men and women play in society are not entirely biologically determined, but instead tend to vary with perceived social and cultural needs. Even when they are putatively justified by, say, appeal to some religious teaching, their roles vary widely – even within the same religious group – over time. In fact, they respond particularly rapidly to secular education. Thus, in seeking to improve women's human rights, much can be done while still respecting and upholding different forms of social organisation. When the author was working in Venezuela in the late 1950s, one of his colleagues commented that 'We won't get anywhere with women's and children's rights until we wipe out Catholicism!' Only a few years later, the greatest social progress in Latin America was being made under the umbrella of liberation theology, preached by Catholic churches and vigorously promoted by nuns who were running literacy campaigns. Within four years of the Cuban revolution, the proportion of Roman Catholics in that country had increased by almost a third, because of its links with social justice.[1]

The fact of the matter is that the more a society is free from exploitation within its own ranks, the harder it is for it to be exploited by outside forces, such as transnational corporations. Marc Lalonde[2] made this point in his landmark document that initiated the health promotion movement.

Women are as diverse a group as men with regard to their interests and such characteristics as age, social status, educational orientation, etc. And obviously we have no basis for assuming that concepts like 'sisterhood' should influence their choices any more than 'brotherhood' does among men. Therefore, in this chapter the author will address the issues of specific groups of women in specific situations, and will deal with specific practices (e.g. female genital mutilation). He will then show how specific violations of women's basic human rights are exacerbated by neoliberal financial globalisation and its agencies, and how these same factors also impede women's attempts to solve their own problems, especially in the LDCs.

Women's health

Health, of course, is the most basic of human rights, as without it one is not in as effective a position to demand or exercise other rights. Many cultural practices that are widely prevalent in the LDCs force women into a situation in which their health is compromised. Many of these practices relate to marriage. In a number of Asian and African cultures, male domination is the norm. As we shall see in Chapter 10, this has a catastrophic impact on the education of girls and women. Consider the marriage issue. Worldwide, the idea that a woman can choose whether or not to marry, and to choose her husband if she does decide to marry is by no means universal. One comes across all kinds of arguments and rationalisations that justify the idea of the girl's father (or both her parents) choosing her husband. However, no one can deny that this disempowers the woman in the relationship from the start.

Her status as a bride has been first and foremost determined by a family policy decision, usually based on the father's concern for the preservation of control over the family and clan financial interests. Moreover, anyone who reads Victorian novels is soon disabused of any belief that 'Europeans' or 'whites' have always found such practices inimical to morality (for example, consider Jane Austen's *Pride and Prejudice*). We have moved away from such practices and beliefs largely because our increasing wealth allowed a freeing up of the exercise of autonomy.

In Zimbabwe, as in many other African countries, the concept of 'lobola' is crucial in both of the major tribes, the Shona and the Ndebele. The main purpose of marriage in those societies is to produce children, the husband's lineage. In order to secure the right to these children, the husband's family needs to pay a 'bride price' (lobola) to the bride's family. It is then incumbent upon the bride to 'justify' her father-in-law's expense by being a 'good' wife. If she does not in fact live up to her husband's expectations, he can kick her out and her father has to return the lobola. Not only does this have a serious impact on the economic circumstances of the woman's parents, but also it has a negative effect on her own prospects. Often, in such cases known to the author, the forsaken bride returns in shame to her own home and village, where she becomes little more than an unpaid domestic servant.[3]

Even if the bride escapes this fate, behaves well and remains with her husband, she is still severely disempowered. She not only has to revere her husband, but is also at the beck and call of her in-laws and, usually at least for some time after the marriage, she acts as a servant in her mother-in-law's house. Above all, however, her duty is to bear children, and not only that – the preference is for boys. The reason for this is that only boys carry on the father's name, whereas girls will have children who carry other men's names. However, ignorance is usually such that many people have the idea that it is the mother who determines the sex of any children she bears. As the reader knows, this is in fact determined by the father's gametes, not those of the mother!

This is one important link with education. Whenever this author has taught biology in the Third World (and even sometimes here!) and has explained the genetic basis of sex determination, the information has been received with great surprise and even hostile doubt. However, without this piece of information, failure to produce a son is blamed on the woman and can result in her family having to return the bride price, and in dissolution of the marriage.

The situation in many Asian countries is not dissimilar, and has a particular resonance in certain Islamic communities. In these contexts, the bride is often told who she is to marry without prior consultation, even if it is to someone whom she particularly dislikes or fears. This even applies to many girls who have grown up and attended school in the USA or the EU. There have been numerous cases of young girls who were just about to finish their secondary schooling being taken 'on holiday' back to their parents' home country and forced to marry someone they barely know. Moreover, if they resist or run away, they can be pursued, badly injured or become the subject of an 'honour killing.'

Often these practices do not violate the prevailing law in the country concerned, and it is only within the last few years that, say, the UK has been aggressive in pursuing the victim's interests in such cases. If the violation is carried out in a country that does not regard it as illegal, there is little that the UK can do except to revoke the British citizenship of the parent or parents. More action is possible if the girl herself is a British citizen, in which case the perpetrators can be indicted by a British court.

Before detailing further instances of violation of women's rights in the less developed world, it is important to keep one thing in mind. It is to the clear financial advantage of many TNCs working under WTO auspices to take full advantage of women's disempowerment. Women often form a very large proportion of the workforce in such foreign-owned plants, and are easily kept in line by their lack of rights outside the workplace.

Early marriage in the LDCs

Even outside the various types of family-arranged and forced marriage, the earlier a young woman marries, the less chance she has of developing a strong sense of personal autonomy or self-worth. Yet in the less developed world it is often routine for women to marry very young and have children. Given the financial traps into which this leads them, they readily become compliant and easily exploited employees in clothing factories, piecework manufacturing, food processing, etc. And this has not yet touched on the illegal sex trade that is always beckoning them from the sideline.

In Nigeria, in 1989, this author was assured that 'by the time a girl is 22 years old, she has passed her sell-by date!' Such social expectations put great pressure on girls to marry and to start bearing children before they know much about life. In the developed countries with their disproportionate proportion of the Earth's money supply, young girls sometimes spend more time cultivating their minds, skills and ideas before having children. In the LDCs, it is estimated that 82 million girls between the ages of 10 and 17 years will be married before their eighteenth birthday.[4] Marriage at an early age jeopardises health and safety, both for the young mother and for her children, in many different ways. It certainly limits their educational opportunities, and frequently leads to physical abuse, along with exploitation in the workplace. As we shall see in Chapter 11, it also renders them much more susceptible to HIV/AIDS, especially if – as is generally the case – their marriage partner is an older man with a long sexual history involving other women.

About 14 million women (not all of them married by any means) between the ages of 15 and 19 years give birth each year. In this age group, complications of pregnancy and childbirth are significant causes of death. Unsafe abortions contribute to this figure. We know that early childbearing is linked to the recurrence of *obstetric fistula*. This painful and socially isolating condition often leads to incontinence in those affected. In addition, throughout the world, teenage pregnancy is positively correlated with low birth weight, poor nutrition (of both mother and child) and anaemia. Furthermore, these mothers have a higher risk of developing cervical cancer late in life.[5] It goes without saying that the grave disadvantages of early sexual activity among girls are strongly linked to such hideous abuses as female genital mutilation and sexual trafficking.

Work of the United Nations Population Fund in the LDCs

The goal of the United Nations Population Fund[a] (UNFPA) is to speed up progress in closing the gender gap in primary and secondary education, and to ensure that by 2015 all children complete primary school at least, with girls having equal access to all levels of education. As this author has pointed out previously,[6] in

Third World nations the view is widely held that if there is not enough money to send all one's children to primary school, the eldest boy should be sent. In fact it would make greater economic sense to send a girl, as it is she who may have children, and her impact on their upbringing and on the community will depend on her level of education. Of course such a choice would not be necessary if global human rights were taken seriously.

The UNFPA is one of the UN organisations that is not approved by some political voices in the USA because it is associated with giving advice on family planning, and this is anathema to many on the Christian Right who support George Bush. The USA has refused to fund organisations that dispense free condoms or information on contraception. However, the UNFPA is one of the most effective organisations in addressing the inequities in women's human rights worldwide. The following details are provided on its website (www.unfpa.org/gender/girls.htm), from which the reader can receive information about its programmes.

The UNFPA has been reaching out to young adults together with UNICEF and the World Health Organization in 13 countries. Specifically, they are anxious to ensure that teenage girls have the same rights as teenage boys. The programme is funded by the UN and is based on six strategies:

1 keeping girls in school until they have completed secondary education
2 providing youth-friendly reproductive health advice and facilities
3 working with religious bodies and other community organisations
4 giving adolescent girls counselling on their rights and appropriate negotiation skills
5 mobilising cross-agency support at all levels of government with regard to adolescent sexual and reproductive health
6 reinforcing the capacity of national governments to engage girls in the social, political and economic life of the country.

The following are some examples of the UNFPA's programme in action.

In the Palestinian Authority, local communities have already benefited from reproductive health education campaigns, including inputs into school curricula. There has also been a close collaboration with local radio, newspapers and other media. The need for easy access to reproductive health services in schools has been stressed. In Senegal, similar initiatives have been undertaken, especially to help 10,000 disadvantaged girls and women to break the cycle of poverty. As well as training girls in income-generating skills, they have been given access to counselling on sexual issues. In Ethiopia, Bangladesh and India, the UNFPA, working with UNICEF, the Population Council and the International Planned Parenthood Federation (IPPF), have started a project to improve social and economic opportunities for teenage girls. They are working to end the practice of childhood marriages, and in particular they are encouraging young people to work as advocates in HIV prevention with local politicians and policy makers.

Women and the human right to water

As was indicated in Chapter 4, the human right to water is basic to all other rights. Denial of this right has a much more profound and immediate impact on women than on any other group. It is usually women who have to fetch water for families in the LDCs, and who have to rely on its being fit for use. In fact, it is in relation to the right of access to water that the impact of neoliberal global finance reflects its hostility to women's rights, through WTO insistence on water privatisation schemes. If, instead of being regarded as a 'human right' per se, water becomes regarded as an 'economic good' or a 'commodity', it can be privatised. This has happened frequently in Africa (*see* Chapter 4). Consider the following example from Kenya's experience, as described by Annabell Waititu.[7]

> In Kenya, a 1999 water policy act recognized water as a human right, and made the government fully responsible for ensuring every citizen access. But a new policy in 2002 defined water as an 'economic good' and called upon consumers to pay for it. The administration of President Mwai Kibaki, which was trying to curry favour with international institutions to increase aid flows, has also supported private sector participation in the water system. A US $ 75 million Privatization and Private Sector Development Project for Kenya is in the World Bank pipeline and it has water privatization as a core objective.
>
> For now, the water systems remain publicly owned in cities, reliability varies, but the quality of piped water is generally good. Overall, however, about 50% of the population in both rural and urban areas lack clean water. They must purchase it from vendors, paying more than 30 times the price of piped supplies. Some draw water from polluted sources, such as wells and springs. Water-borne diseases are believed to be responsible for most children's deaths.
>
> While women play a critical role in the water sector, they are rarely integrated into actual practice or policy. Some women are taking matters into their own hands, forming local associations that work with municipalities to ensure that piped-water points are established within their reach. They have mobilized neighbourhoods, municipalities and other partners to build water tanks, and have generated funds locally to pay for them.

There are many other examples that may be cited, but suffice it to say that most human rights advocates regard water as a particularly critical component of gender equality and the empowerment of women. Thus privatisation of water intensifies gender inequalities. Because household use of water does not generate income directly, the traditional economic indicators fail to capture it. Furthermore, women on a low income who are facing time and energy constraints are often obliged to make use of lower-quality water (e.g. from contaminated ground, close at hand), and thus family health is threatened. Their lack of education also conspires to render them unaware of the risks. This is especially worrying in view of the fact that 80% of all illnesses are transmitted by contaminated water. The author has often worked in communities in which girls are routinely kept away from school in order to make the necessary daily long journey to obtain safe water. Travelling such long distances, alone, puts them at greatly increased risk of physical violence.

In general, this privatisation of water supplies is part and parcel of the structural adjustment policies (SAPs), which are imposed as conditionalities on IMF loans. Again this clearly illustrates how the exploitation of women, and denial of their human rights, does redound to the benefit of First World corporate interests – even though such UN agencies as the IMF and the WTO may be the intermediaries! The global trend towards the privatisation of water therefore increases the assault on women's rights, and thereby disempowers communities. When water is a 'public' provision, women (as major users of it) have some say in democratic regimes as to how it is supplied. However, corporations have no such obligation, and public access to information about corporations is restricted.

Indeed, the exploitation of women is such a good source of income that it is not entirely restricted to the Third World. Consider a situation in Detroit, USA, where women's groups organised in 2003 to oppose a major water privatisation scheme there. They are still at it![8]

Genital mutilation

In speaking of women's rights it is usual to refer only to *female genital mutilation (FGM)*, but for completeness and to put it in context, there is also male genital mutilation. Circumcision of boys was, until recently, increasingly regarded as unnecessary and a violation of their human rights. And in a very few societies (e.g. some Australian Aborigine cultures) it involves much more intrusive cutting and far more pain than we normally associate with the term 'circumcision.' Moreover, the procedure is not usually performed in the Aborigine context until the boy has almost reached puberty, so he will certainly have a clear memory of the procedure and be much more likely to suffer psychological trauma after the event than if it had been done when he was 8 days old. However, even the routine western technique of performing circumcision on boys barely a week old, and under proper medical conditions, became widely condemned, and there were also claims that it can have adverse psychological effects later in life.

Revised views on male circumcision

As mentioned above, there are some who argue that male circumcision in babyhood may be psychologically traumatic, but the findings of recently published research may herald a resurgence in the practice for medical reasons. At the Sixteenth International HIV/AIDS Conference held in Toronto, Canada, in August 2006, papers were presented which indicated that rates of male circumcision and of HIV/AIDS infection are inversely correlated.

Indeed, some of these findings were published in *The Times of Zambia*[9] on the eve of the Conference. Both local and international research indicated that, in Africa, wherever male circumcision rates exceeded 80%, HIV prevalence fell below 10%. It is estimated that performing male circumcision throughout Africa could avert up to 5.7 million HIV infections by 2026. A South African study conducted last year suggested that male circumcision reduced the HIV acquisition rate in males by 60%. Of course, such findings have to be treated cautiously. Circumcised men are not immune to HIV infection, and in the social context of restricted women's rights and male promiscuity, infection remains a fundamental problem to be overcome.

However, female genital mutilation is a much more serious act of violence, for three reasons.

1 It is done when the child is old enough to remember it. I worked with a highly educated male Kenyan colleague in 1983, who one day commented that he would have to be absent for a while because he had to go home to his village to circumcise his 6-year-old daughter. I was surprised, as this man had received all of his postgraduate training (none of it in health-related disciplines, I must add!) at top-rated universities in the USA and Australia in sociology. I therefore asked him both what training he had received to perform such a procedure, and why he was doing it. In response he explained that, as Headsman in his village, his daughter would be disgraced if he didn't do it, and her chances of getting married could be compromised. He also explained that he had received no training, but none was required 'because women of the village would hold her down!' In answer to the question 'why', he explained that the procedure would prevent his daughter, in later life when she was married, from 'jumping the fence' (i.e. having casual sex on the side): 'She will always remember the pain.' He argued that it was a cultural matter and that all of the women in her circle had had it done, and that when the initial pain had subsided after a few days, she would feel proud of having had it done.
2 FGM is much more extensive, in surgical terms, than the male equivalent.
3 Even when done with a sterilised Exacto blade, there is a far greater risk of post-operative infection when it is not performed in aseptic conditions or by medically qualified individuals.

Female genital mutilation (FGM)

This procedure is also called 'female circumcision', but that term for it is more often used by people who advocate the practice, whereas the term 'FGM' is generally used by those who oppose it. The procedure has no medical justification whatsoever. There are four main types of FGM.[10]

1 *'Sunna' circumcision* consists of the removal of the tip of the clitoris and/or the prepuce (the covering of the clitoris).
2 *Clitoridectomy/excision* consists of the removal of the entire clitoris (both the prepuce and the glans), and the removal of the entire adjacent labia.
3 *Infibulation* consists of the removal of the clitoris and the adjacent labia (majora and minora), followed by stitching together of the scraped sides of the vulva across the vagina. A small opening is retained to allow the passage of urine and menstrual blood.
4 *Unclassified* includes other forms of FGM, such as:

   • pricking, piercing or incision of the clitoris and/or labia
   • stretching of the clitoris and/or labia
   • cauterisation by burning of the clitoris and surrounding tissue
   • scraping of tissue surrounding the vaginal orifice or cutting of the vagina
   • introduction of corrosive substances or herbs into the vagina to cause bleeding, or for the purpose of tightening or narrowing it.

The majority of mutilations (80–85%) are of types 1 and 2, while infibulation (type 3) accounts for 15%.[11]

In 1997, the World Health Organization estimated that about 2 million girls a year face this procedure, usually between the ages of 4 and 8 years.[10] Most of these are from 28 countries in Africa, some Asian countries, the Middle East, and immigrant communities in the EU and the USA. In the African countries of Djibouti, Eritrea, Sierra Leone, Somalia and Sudan, around 90% of women are estimated to have been so treated.[11] The actual procedure varies widely between countries and also according to ethnic group, area (urban or rural) and socio-economic status. In the LDCs it is performed by all kinds of people, usually older women, and with instruments ranging from a piece of broken glass to some type of proper blade. In urban areas, and certainly in the developed world, it is usually done in hospitals under medical supervision.

Women whom this author has interviewed about the procedure universally described it as 'terrifying' and 'agonising' when not done under medical supervision, but as 'rather like having an appendix out' when done in hospital. However, almost all of them claimed that it was 'a good thing', and many made comments like 'I would not have been a full woman without it.' None of these women could cite a 'real' advantage. Some of them cited medical advantages, but these had no real validity. Added to this is the fact that female circumcision is far more likely to have long-term after-effects, including the following:

- difficulty in passing menstrual fluid, especially in cases of infibulation. Partial retention of menses can lead to a foul smell and infection in its own right
- infection (at least local) – a very common consequence of all four forms of FGM. Such infection is almost certain if the procedure is not performed with a sterile instrument under aseptic conditions
- death as an immediate result of FGM is not common, but is frequent enough for a number of people to whom I have spoken to recall cases
- persistent infections lasting for several weeks, with episodes of fever, etc., are quite common
- collateral damage to surrounding tissues
- urinary incontinence
- psychological trauma.

While working in communities in which FGM is practised, I became aware of what people said were the positive effects. In discussing these with women, I would invariably acknowledge their beliefs but would also point out that until only recently views in the developed-world countries about the 'benefits' of male circumcision were being questioned – as far back as the 1970s. Some Muslim people cite religious reasons, as some people in the First World still do about male circumcision, but these views are not universally accepted by Muslims, Jews or Christians. The religious arguments do not persuade most Muslims, and it seems to be more of a geographical issue, being common among Muslims in Africa but not among those in the Middle East. My view is that the practice of female circumcision will die out in the face of more widespread education, and more widespread access to such means of communication as computers, a point on which I shall elaborate in Chapter 10.

Iron her breasts to keep men away

An even more outrageous form of violence against women is the practice of ironing the breasts of girls as they begin to mature. This is every bit as brutal as it sounds, and only seemed to come to light on a BBC World Service radio broad-cast at 3am on 23 June 2006. This terribly painful form of disfigurement is inflicted on the girl by her mother (or another close relative), and is done with a domestic hot iron or with hot stones. The poor girl is laid on her back and held down while her budding breasts are systematically flattened. The unbelievable details of this practice were released on 13 June 2006 by the Inter Press Service of Johannesburg.[12] As far as this author has been able to ascertain, the practice is confined to Cameroon.

Gender violence as supportive of male power

It is obvious that a great deal of gender violence arises as a means of securing and maintaining male domination. This is implicit even in some religious contexts, in which women are expected to endure all manner of discomfort, inconvenience and restrictions on their freedom in order to 'protect' them from male sexual assault. The implication is that men's sexual appetite cannot be controlled by themselves, so the onus is on women to protect themselves against it. This idea must go way back in history, as one finds it expressed even in pre-Judaic litera-ture, in which the 'female' figure is presented as the beguiling temptress, an agent of the forces of darkness.

This is also consistent with the extremely high incidence of violation of women's rights during wars, even when such crimes are serving no military pur-pose. Military action has always been associated with strongly phallic symbols (e.g. lances, swords, rifles, etc.), and it is extraordinary how persistent this 'Freudian' symbolism is. Without much conscious thought, and certainly with no literary or artistic knowledge in most cases, it very quickly becomes experienced overtly by male soldiers in battle. In most military occupations, it is women and girl civilians who suffer the most.

However, war is of course a crucially profitable activity for multinational investment. Another important profit-making activity for TNCs is that of the extractive industries. As the dominant players in financing large-scale mining, the Bretton Woods institutions are again implicated in large-scale violation of women's rights. It is therefore no coincidence that women in the less developed world play such a prominent role in organised opposition to major mining proj-ects in their own countries. Of course, some mining activity in the LDCs has been going on for centuries and has become 'culturally sustainable' in the communi-ties concerned. For instance, the Igorot people in the Philippines have mined and traded gold with Chinese merchants for the last 700 years. Likewise, historical records show that since the ninth century, African traders from the southern areas of the continent have been engaged in mining, smelting, and trading as far afield as India. These smaller-scale mining activities have not been particularly associated with gender violence. However, larger and more recent mining proj-ects have been implicated in this way.

Most of what is mined in the Third World by the TNCs is used for trade on the world market, and this was a principal mechanism for integrating the Third World communities involved into the global economy. Most of these projects have been financed, since the 1970s, by the IMF, with their SAPs as condition-alities. It is principally women and children whose rights have been sacrificed as a consequence, due to the SAP requirement that government-funded social services (education, healthcare, etc.) be cut. However, another aspect of such mining involves what is referred to as the 'Regalian Doctrine.'

The Regalian Doctrine applies in most LDCs, and in effect gives the government the right to take control of any land under which valuable mining resources have been found. The TNC mining companies, being well staffed with the requisite geological expertise, are quick to discover such deposits and to agree lucrative deals with the local governments concerned. This leads to the swift dispossession of entire communities (homes, schools, etc.), with little or no recompense. This has a particular impact on families in general, and often on discrete ethnic communities, indigenous tribal groupings, etc.,[13] as will be discussed in Chapter 13.

Generally speaking, the impact of large-scale community upheaval, whether it is caused by war, mining or even natural disasters (such as earthquakes, hurricanes, etc.) has a potentially grievous impact on reproductive health. Women and children account for more than 75% of refugees and displaced people at risk from such events worldwide. Women of reproductive age represent about 25% of such at-risk populations, and about 20% of these women are likely to be pregnant. In addition, many women, when forced to flee, were poor at the time and were therefore particularly vulnerable to sexual exploitation and violence.[14]

Trafficking of women

In societies in which women and girls are significantly excluded from normal human rights, they are naturally more prone to exploitation of all kinds. For instance, when this author was working in Nepal in 1997, he was aware of a steady trafficking of young girls – some as young as 10 or 11 years – by groups sending them to India, Pakistan, the EU and even the USA. The Indian subcontinent was by far the commonest destination.

However, the trade is astonishingly wide, varied and profitable. It has always been multiracial, and recently, with a number of less wealthy eastern European nations now having access to the EU, it has involved thousands of white European women and girls. Gender aside, it is another example of the tyranny of poverty. If MDG 1 (the halving of global poverty) was to be realised by 2015, almost certainly the trafficking of women would be dealt a mortal blow. The trade in women and girls is very often run by the same organisations that deal internationally in the drugs trade. In that context, women are no more than a commodity like any other item – a clear reflection of the immorality that is made possible and indeed likely by the persistence of global inequalities. And, as with any large-scale inhuman and illegal activity, social upheaval and war commonly accompany it.

For example, in January 2001, the media reported a protracted pitched battle between Thai, Burmese (Myanmarese) and ethnic insurgents which claimed over 100 lives on both sides of the Thai–Burma border. The town at the centre of the conflict was Tachilek, which is in the infamous Golden Triangle in Burma, and is best known as the major conduit for opium and methamphetamines from Burma to outlets in the EU and the USA. Consistent with its generally unsavoury reputation, it also has a Thai-owned casino and a thriving black market in everything from pirate DVDs to tiger skins, Burmese antiques – and women and girls.

The latter commodity has only increased and become much more tightly organised in the last decade, but when the author was in Thailand in 1983 and briefly entered Tachilek, the sex trade was constantly brought to his notice by men coming up to him and whispering hoarsely (in Thai) 'phuying – suay maak' ('girls – very beautiful'). Burma, of course, is at present run by a corrupt and violent military dictatorship (that prefers the country to be called Myanmar), and it is not surprising to learn that in 2001 about 65% of Burma's wealth came from such illicit sources.[15]

In the same article, a physician working for the NGO World Vision states:

> There are a great many prostitutes going back and forth between the border towns for sex work, largely supported by visiting tourists from wealthy countries. At least 30% of those crossing the line are sex workers. We cannot know exactly what this implies for the transmission of HIV/AIDS, but we do know that 12% of pregnant women in the border town of Kawthaung (in Thailand) are HIV positive, compared to 7% in Ramong (on the Burma side). The HIV rate therefore must be much higher among the sex workers in Kawthaung. Entire towns are now known primarily for their sex business. Most customers are truck drivers carrying goods – and AIDS – from Thailand and China.[15]

Variety and scope of sex trafficking

Many varieties of trafficking exist, but by far the largest involves sexual exploitation. There is even a flourishing industry in mail-order brides! Another variety involves exporting workers, usually as domestic servants, so that they can send a portion of their wages back home. These workers often live in opulent houses, but invisibly, with few comforts and little outside contact. Until recently, most of these women came from LDCs such as those in the Pacific islands, Africa, Southeast Asia, etc., but now a sizeable number come from the former communist republics of eastern Europe.

Typically, they come from either rural areas or urban slums, sometimes as 'tourist workers' or as victims of kidnap in order to be forced into sexual slavery. Many are sold, and in fact in some countries, as we shall see, they are even sold in markets in broad daylight. To call them 'women' is a misnomer, for many are very young, between 10 and 15 years of age. Some have not yet started to menstruate and have no idea what sexual activity involves.

These girls are purchased for US$ 400 to US$ 800 and are told that they must stay in the brothel where they end up until their price has been paid for. At most, they receive only 20% of the money that is charged for their services, and they are routinely cheated even on this. Yet even when they eventually are 'free', they are still victims because they are often in the country illegally and their passports have been stolen. If they do manage to get back home, they are often stigmatised for life.[16]

The number of women and children who are being exploited in this way is increasing exponentially. It is estimated that sex trafficking involves anywhere between one and two million a year. At a Southeast Asian women's organisation in 1991 it was estimated that 30 million women had been trafficked worldwide since 1975. Japan alone receives more than 100,000 such 'sex workers.' Nepal 'exports' thousands of women a year to India, and similarly from Myanmar

(Burma) to Thailand. During 1993, 200,000 women were sent from Bangladesh to Pakistan. In the same way, women from China are turning up in Thailand, women from Latin America and the Caribbean are ending up in the USA, and so on. In addition, a lucrative 'internal' market is flourishing in many nations.[17]

The above data are derived from Judith Mirkinson's authoritative research, and as she points out, the entire terrible trade has always relied on the preservation of vast global inequalities in wealth. That is why it has increased so dramatically as the gap in human rights equity between the less developed and the developed countries has widened.

Moreover, it cannot be assumed that the good will of ordinary people can impose any kind of moral check on this. Inequity always creates exploitation – even of children – once they become commodities. Children are being sold at ever younger ages. The same obscene difference in wealth between the First World and the Third World ensures this, and accelerates demand, as sex tourism allows more and more people from wealthy countries to visit poor countries and make use of their women and children. Some developed countries (e.g. the UK) have finally made it a criminal offence in their home country if one of their citizens commits abroad what would be regarded as a sexual offence at home.

One of the rationalisations (very prevalent in the Middle East and parts of Asia and Africa) for sexual abuse of under-age children is a belief that intercourse with a virgin child can cure HIV/AIDS and other sexually transmitted diseases. Using this justification, children as young as 8 years are now being provided globally for these services. The figures are appalling. There are around 800,000 child prostitutes in Thailand, around 400,000 in India, around 250,000 in Brazil and around 60,000 in the Philippines. About 20,000 children are shipped from Burma to Thailand each year for this trade. Because their internal vaginal tissues are not yet fully mature, children are much more vulnerable to HIV/AIDS. Around 25% of child prostitutes are HIV positive, and 50% of prostitutes under the age of 18 years in Thailand have contracted HIV.[18]

All of the above highlights the importance of education in promoting human rights. The abuse of women and children for profit is happening not only in LDCs but also increasingly in the developed countries.

Mail-order brides and domestic workers

The gradual penetration of neoliberal globalisation of finance has now undermined the less developed world so thoroughly that it has greatly facilitated the exploitation of women. As this author stated in an earlier book,[19] 'Take away the resources of a country, and the people will soon follow.' Verticalisation of health and educational services in a poor country to facilitate its economic restructuring along WTO lines, or to meet IMF conditionalities, virtually guarantees that thousands of vulnerable people will be desperate to chase the chance to make a good living all the way to a well-heeled First World country. The UK is an especially favoured target, for a number of reasons.

Out of this desperation has mushroomed a highly lucrative business – mail-order brides. Starting in the 1980s, advertisements for this business began to appear in respectable newspapers in London, New York and elsewhere, and it did look innocent enough. However, these ads represent megabucks. By 1997, there were about 50,000 mail-order brides (MOBs) from the Philippines alone in the USA. As Judith Mirkinson[20] points out:

> The women are often isolated and scared; many become virtual slaves in their own homes. Sometimes these 'marriages' work out. Many times they don't, and sometimes there are disastrous consequences. Women have been tortured and killed. Some men use their wives as prostitutes or for pornography. Clearly, not all the husbands are psychotic, but the incidence of violence against mail-order brides is extremely high. The agencies that recruit and then sell the brides are not sleazy hole-in-the-wall places. They're legitimate businesses. One of the biggest, Cherry Blossom, which has its headquarters in Hawaii, is run by a Princeton University MBA.

As Mirkinson points out, one defence against this type of exploitation is to lobby media outlets to get rid of the advertisements. She quotes the example of *Harper's Magazine*, a very upmarket New York publication. It stopped running the ads as a result of a letter-writing campaign.

The situation facing domestic workers from the LDCs can be just as bad. During the first of the Gulf Wars (the one to prevent Iraq from occupying Kuwait), the media broadcast an account of how the Spanish Embassy in Kuwait was besieged by hundreds of Filipino women seeking shelter because they feared for their lives. Thousands of them had been penned up in wealthy Kuwait homes as virtual slaves, but with the invasion they found themselves threatened with rape by both Kuwaiti and Iraqi soldiers.

During the early 1970s, when the IMF and the World Bank became really heavily involved in loans to LDCs, these two organisations drew up a scheme whereby the Philippine government could generate income by exporting armies of its young men as construction workers and of its young women as domestic workers. For that purpose they even set up a Philippine Overseas Employment Agency. By the late 1970s, the vast majority of Filipinos working abroad were women, and not all of these were 'domestic workers.' The numbers involved were huge. To quote Mirkinson, for 1997 they were as follows:[21]

- 75,000 prostituted women in Japan
- 50,000 maids in Singapore
- 50,000 domestics/prostituted women in Hong Kong
- 75,000 domestics in England
- 50,000 domestics in Spain
- 75,000 domestics in Italy
- 50,000 in Germany
- 150,000 in the Middle East.

The IMF was not unduly worried that the conditions of employment almost always contravened their human rights. Some of the luckier women ended up in Canada, where within two years, if they were married or lived in their employer's residence, they could gain residency rights. However, in Saudi Arabia and Kuwait a woman's passport was immediately taken from her by the Immigration authorities, and in Singapore and Hong Kong the woman's employer held her passport. In most cases these women have no redress for their bad treatment, and there is no supervision of their living or working conditions.

Concluding comment

In doing the research for this chapter, the author has confronted statistics for and accounts of institutional and episodic treatment of women and girls that have left him shaken. Such material emphasises the importance not only of meeting the Millennium Development Goals themselves, but also of being tireless in our pursuit of full global human rights as outlined in the UN Charter. There can be no national basis for addressing the issue. It must be international. The next chapter deals with the universal right to schooling, at least to the level of literacy and numeracy. But that, of course, depends first on the assurance of universal women's rights.

The issues dealt with in this chapter are enormous, and merit much more attention, and by people better qualified to address them. In my view, the task could not really be carried out by a man, however well intentioned and informed. In closing this chapter, allow me to quote from a speech given by Charlotte Bunch,[22] Executive Director of the Centre for Women's Global Leadership, in March 2004.

> It is to be expected that global inequalities in wealth will, if they persist, lead to global inequalities in access to medical treatment, information and empowerment. Worldwide, women remain the poorest of the poor. In fact, the gap between women's empowerment has increased between the developed and less developed countries. Development experts are unanimous in the view that improving the status of women is the key to national development, but much more needs to be done about it than is currently the case, and many trends are working against it.

Privatisation – for example, of social services, health and education – impacts most adversely on women and children. Neoliberal financial globalisation seems to fit in perfectly with old-fashioned patriarchal attitudes and fundamentalist 'traditionalism.' They are mutually supportive, and before any progress with regard to equity in human rights can be made, that nexus must be broken.

References

1 MacDonald T. *Making a New People: revolutionary development of Cuba's educational system.* Vancouver: New Star Books; 1983. p. 19.
2 Lalonde M. *A Perspective on the Health of all Canadians.* Ottawa: Government Publications; 1974.
3 MacDonald T. *Third World Health: hostage to First World wealth.* Oxford: Radcliffe Publishing; 2005. p. 171.
4 United Nations Population Fund (UNPF). *Promoting Gender Equality: girls and adolescents;* www.unfpa.org/gender/girls/htm (accessed 23 June 2006).
5 Ibid., p. 10.
6 MacDonald T (2005), op. cit., p. 86.
7 Waititu A. *Diverting the Flow: gender rights and water privatisation.* New York: Women's Environment Development Organization; 2006. p. 4.
8 Taylor M. *United States Returning to Back Door.* New York: Women's Environment Development Organization; 2006. p. 9.
9 Mwendabai D. Male circumcision receiving attention. *The Times of Zambia (Ndola),* 14 August 2006, p. 1.

10 World Health Organization. *Fact Sheet on FGM;* www.who.int/inf-fs/en/fact153.htm (accessed 21 June 2006).

11 World Health Organization. *Estimated Prevalence of FGM in Africa;* http://anmesty.org/aiblib/intcam/femgen/fym1.htm (accessed 23 June 2006).

12 Yaouode ST. *Cameroon: An Unwelcome Gift of God.* Johannesburg: Inter Press Service. 13 June 2006. www.allafrica.com/stories/20060614007.html (accessed 16 June 2006).

13 Tauli-Corpuz V. *The globalization of mining and its impact and challenges for women.* Paper given at the International Conference on Women and Mining held at Baguio City, Philippines, 20–23 January 1997. www.twnside.org.sg/title/chal-cn.htm (accessed 23 June 2006).

14 *Women in Emergency Situations.* UNFPA Population Issues; www.unfpa.org/gender/emergency.htm (accessed 23 June 2006).

15 Lawrence N. Sex for export. *The Irrawaddy,* 2001; **9;** www.irrawaddy.org/database/2001/vol19.2/sexexport.htm (accessed 23 June 2006).

16 *The Global Trafficking of Women;* http://feminism.eserver.org/gender/sex-work/trafficking-of-women.tx (accessed 23 June 2006).

17 Mirkinson J. *Red Light/Green Light: the global trafficking of women.* San Francisco, CA: Breakthrough: Journal of the Prairie Fire Organizing Committee; 1994. p. 6.

18 HIV/AIDS Council. *Child Prostitution and AIDS;* www.thebody.com/whatis/sexwork.htm/1

19 MacDonald T. *Third World Health: hostage to First World wealth.* Oxford: Radcliffe Publishing; 2005. p. 14.

20 Mirkinson J, op. cit., p. 7.

21 Mirkinson J, op. cit., pp. 7–8.

22 Bunch C. *Where are we in 2004?* Speech given at US Committee for UNIFEM Lunch, UN Headquarters, New York, 4 March 2004.

Endnote

[a] The United Nations Population Fund (UNPF) has only had that name since 1987, when UNESCO changed it from the original 1989 name of United Nations Fund for Population Activities (UNFPA). The author has noticed that many references to the UNPF still call it the UNFPA.

Chapter 9

In defence of children and their rights

Who are the children?

Before looking at the issues in broader terms, let us consider the technical question 'What is a child?' Under Article 1 of the UN Convention on the Rights of the Child (1989), a child is defined as:

> ... every human being below the age of 18 years unless, under the law applicable to the child, majority is attained earlier.[1]

Even in older democracies, where the rule of law is traditionally well established, this can give rise to anomalies. For instance, in the UK, until recently, there were differences between the age at which one was legally allowed to engage in sexual activity according to one's sexual preferences, and the ages at which one could drink in a pub or buy alcohol, fight for one's country, vote, marry or face criminal trial in an 'adult' court. So the issue, if looked at globally, is far from clear.

However, 18 years of age is now generally accepted as the end of childhood. In fact, since the UN Convention on the Rights of the Child was introduced, the International Labour Organization (ILO) has introduced its Convention Number 182 on the Worst Forms of Child Labour. This categorically states that all individuals aged below 18 years should be regarded as children.

Childhood and unknown rights

The word 'child' immediately implies two things – vulnerability and the need for advocacy. Humans have the longest period of juvenility of any species, both in terms of absolute number of years and in terms of the proportion of total lifespan. This increases with progress in elaborating technological advances and in intellectual advance of the species, because more and more time has to be added to children's period of initiation into adulthood before they can cope and survive optimally. Thus in eighteenth-century England, it was not uncommon for a person to have left home and school and to be independently employed before the age of 12 years. In the case of males this frequently meant that a boy did not reach puberty until he had already established himself as independent of his parents. In that sense the actual link between active sexuality and the end of dependency on adults for survival was pretty much as it is among other mammals.

In many parts of the less developed world this is indeed still the case, but not in the technologically advanced nations, and the reasons for this are obvious. Children growing up in the USA or the EU, Australia, Canada or a few other First World countries can no longer depend on the availability of unskilled work. They have to, at the very minimum, complete both primary and secondary schooling, and generally quite a bit more, before throwing themselves on to the labour market. This introduces a whole new range of psychological stressors that were largely unknown even a century ago, such as having to live at home, being restricted socially, meeting the demands of arbitrarily imposed authority (at school) without payment for the work done, and so on. In general, of course, we find that the stress is worthwhile, because of the much greater scope for freedom, experience and control that such a long apprenticeship usually confers.

However, this difference in social psychology between the developed and less developed world itself further entrenches the equity gap that the Millennium Development Goals (MDGs) are designed to narrow. If we are to insist on global human rights for children, we have much to do with regard to the issues of *vulnerability* and *advocacy*. Both imply the need for vastly improved protection, even though the recipient may – due to his or her juvenility – not appreciate the reason for it. Children are rarely in a position to demand the rights that are due them, even if they know that they have such rights and it is up to legal sanctions to define and defend those rights. Each culture and nation goes about this task in a different way, but the UN's mandate has included setting an international standard. MDGs 2, 3, 4 and 5 all converge on this, for in order to protect the child we certainly need to protect the mother.

UN Convention on the Rights of the Child

Out of these considerations, then, was formed the UN Convention on the Rights of the Child (CRC), as formally defined in 1990. It has been adopted in every country in the world with the exception of Somalia and the USA. Protecting children from unfair employment practices by TNCs in the less developed world would run rather counter to the corporate interests in profiting from such TNCs. Because of this, Somalia has been at war almost continuously since 1990.[1] That may just be coming to an end, and possibly it will not be long before Somalia can be persuaded to sign up to the CRC.

Four main principles undergird the Convention. A child has the right:

1   to survival and development
2   not to be discriminated against purely on the grounds of his or her incomplete development
3   to be informed about, and to participate in, any decisions that affect him or her
4   to the assumption that anything which is done to him or her can demonstrably be shown to be in his or her best interests.

Despite the two non-signatories, the Convention on the Rights of the Child ranks among the most widely accepted of international conventions. However, it has been extremely difficult to implement, especially the principle regarding the 'best interests of the child.' Without question, poverty is a major barrier to enforcement, but the Convention can be used to assess a country's human rights record. It can certainly be used as a criterion to evaluate the types of care that are made available for vulnerable children. For instance, orphans do not generally thrive so well in institutional settings as in surrogate families. This allows countries to be advised when making such provisions. Institutional care can be severely criticised, in particular because research has shown that it arrests psychological development and socialisation, can prevent optimal levels of participation in care, and can promote stigma and discrimination. Even nominal adherence to the Convention can formalise issues such as birth registration and inheritance rights, and it can provide a legal basis for preventing sexual abuse and child labour. Indeed, on the basis of the Convention, a global strategies framework to cover such issues was drawn up in 2004.

This framework has been particularly effective in providing an international basis for protecting orphans and other children who are rendered vulnerable as a result of HIV/AIDS.[2] This issue will be discussed in greater detail in Chapter 11.

Rights of the children implies the right to safe maternity

As stated earlier, implicit in defining the rights of infants are the rights of their mothers. Yet, worldwide, one woman dies every minute because of problems during pregnancy or childbirth. The magnitude of such an appalling statistic is hard to overstate. It also illustrates most spectacularly the global inequity in maternity, and almost perfectly correlates with the poverty–wealth axis. The vast majority of these deaths are avoidable, but if current trends continue, the target of cutting maternal deaths by 27% by 2015 will not be met.[3]

Governments in the developing world could transform the situation simply by increasing the aid that they give to less developed countries (LDCs), but most do not even achieve the modest goal of 0.7% of their GNP. It would cost US$ 4 billion extra each year to save 500,000 lives. The number of preventable maternal deaths is huge but, unlike sudden and dramatic natural disasters such as earthquakes or tsunamis, it doesn't generate headlines. As we know, the international community has pledged to meet the eight MDGs by 2015, and that includes the commitment to reduce maternal mortality to meet their obligations. Breaking these promises is costing lives.

Key statistical definitions

The issue of infant mortality is complex because different countries have often defined the key indicators differently. Since 1990, the World Health Organization has used the following definitions, and most countries have fallen into line with regard to these.

1   *Infant mortality* is the death of infants within the first year of life. In the LDCs, the leading causes of infant mortality are dehydration and waterborne diseases. In the First World, the major causes of infant mortality are congenital malformation, infection and sudden infant death syndrome (SIDS). Infant mortality can be subdivided as follows.

   - *Perinatal mortality* refers to deaths between the age of fetal viability (defined as 28 weeks of pregnancy or 1,000 g body weight) and the end of the 7th day of life.
   - *Neonatal mortality* refers to deaths in the first 27 days of life.
   - *Postnatal death* refers to deaths between the ages of 28 days and 1 year.

2   *Child mortality* refers to deaths within the first 5 years of life.

The basic definitions now allow us to define a crucial measure that is critical for understanding any discourse about healthcare in children, namely the *infant mortality rate (IMR)*. This is defined as the number of newborns who die before the age of 1 year, divided by the number of live births during that year. It is important to realise that the IMR is generally regarded by people working in the field to be the best predictor of a state's failure or success.[4]

IMR is expressed as the number of live newborns who die before 1 year of age per 1,000 live births, so that IMRs from different countries can be compared. A good reference source for the most recent IMRs as well as the under-five mortality rates (U5MRs) is the UNICEF publication, *The State of the World's Children* (http://unicef.org/publications/index_18108.html). For example, the worst U5MR is 284 (that is, 28% of all children who are born die before they reach the age of 5 years), in Sierra Leone. The 29 countries with the highest U5MRs are all in Africa. The U5MR of the USA is 8 per 1,000 live births, and there are 31 countries with lower U5MRs, although some of them use a less stringent definition of mortality than does the USA. Sweden has the lowest U5MR, at 3 per 1,000 live births.

Critical areas of need

Women in sub-Saharan Africa contribute much more than their share to maternal mortality. They account for only 14% or so of the world's women, but around 50% of maternal mortality. Mortality during pregnancy does occur in developed-world nations, but at a much lower rate. For instance, in the UK the rate is only 1 death per 500 pregnancies, whereas in Ethiopia the rate is 1 in 14 pregnancies – more than 30 times worse. In fact, in much of Africa and South Asia, pregnancy and childbirth constitute the single largest cause of death among women of childbearing age.[5]

As was suggested in Chapter 8, high mortality rates during pregnancy can be traced in many instances to violation of women's rights under the UN Charter. Ultimately, however, they can generally be traced back to deep-rooted prejudicial attitudes towards women. Women have restricted access to schooling and healthcare, and they are compelled to do a disproportionate share of very heavy work (collecting water, cleaning, etc.). They have little impact on decision-making processes and they are also disadvantaged with regard to access to food. All of this is combined with poor healthcare services. There is a lack of trained staff and of appropriate drugs and personal charges for most treatments. While by no means an adequate response, one requirement is an immediate increase in funds from the developed to the less developed world.[6]

Unfortunately, methods of calculating IMR vary widely from one country to another, which makes comparisons difficult. The WHO definition of a live birth is that the baby breathes independently, exhibits muscle movement on testing for it, and has a heartbeat. However, some babies that survive are unable to breathe at birth and have to be stimulated to do so. Yet in some countries (e.g. Japan) such a baby would be considered to be dead.

For the world as a whole, and for both the LDCs and the developed countries, the IMR declined between 1960 and 2001. The world IMR declined from 198 in 1960 to 83 in 2001, but the IMR still remains much higher in the less developed world. In 2001, the IMR for the poorest countries was about 10 times that for the 8 wealthiest countries. The IMR in the poorest countries is around 17 times higher than that in the wealthiest. Furthermore, although reductions in IMR have been achieved in the less developed world, they do not make up for the reductions made during the same period in the developed world. This reflects differences in wealth and spending power to access the necessary basic healthcare and technology.[7]

Table 9.1 gives a clear indication of the gap that we are addressing.

Table 9.1 The five countries with the highest and the five countries with the lowest IMRs in 2006

Rank	Country	Infant mortality rate (deaths/1,000 live births)
1	Angola	187.49
2	Afghanistan	163.07
3	Sierra Leone	162.55
4	Liberia	161.99
5	Mozambique	130.79
222	Iceland	3.31
223	Japan	3.26
224	Hong Kong, SAR, PRC	3.31
225	Sweden	2.77
226	Singapore	2.29

Remediation of such inequities would cost surprisingly little. For instance, the cost of providing basic services for mothers and infants would come to only about US$ 3.00 per person in LDCs. This year (in 2006), 63,000 women in Ethiopia, Mozambique, Tanzania and Uganda will die as a result of obstetric problems. The kind of basic healthcare that could prevent around 80% of these deaths would cost only about US$ 700 per life saved. For most LDCs, US$ 3.00 per head would involve an overwhelmingly large increase in funding for health. For instance, in Ethiopia and Mozambique the total annual spending on health in 2004 amounted to US$ 2.70 per person. This situation definitely calls for large inflows of cash.[8]

For this reason, the nations of the developed world have a moral obligation to see that the MDGs are met. In 2002, the Commission on Macroeconomics and Health, established under the auspices of the World Health Organization, estimated that adequate maternal healthcare would probably require around US$ 4 billion extra each year.[9] Such spending would save about 5 million lives over the next 9 years.

The cost that this would impose on the countries of the developed world is almost trivial – about 1% of the GDP for the OECD (Organization for Economic Cooperation and Development) countries. This is equivalent to about 2 days per year of military spending by the G8 only. Moreover, such aid had already been promised as far back as 1963. At that time, the G7 nations promised to increase their aid to equal 0.7% of their national incomes. If they did reach just that promised level, it would raise an 'additional' US$ 176 billion! This would be sufficient to achieve broad and rapid progress on a number of other MDGs as well.[10]

Infant malnutrition

A major factor in the promotion of infant malnutrition in the less developed world has been the proliferation of TNCs marketing breast-milk substitutes there. The author has addressed this issue extensively in an earlier book.[11] Despite various attempts to prevent the problem on the part of UN agencies, such as the World Health Organization, it still persists. Over the last three or four decades, there has been a dramatic increase in the number of TNCs, and their activities have been increasingly difficult for small countries to regulate because of WTO pressure to maximise free trade. So far, no effective laws have emerged at the international level to control TNCs or hold them to account. Various 'voluntary' or 'self-regulation' agreements between the industries and the governments concerned seem to be regarded as adequate.

This tendency is apparently supported by two beliefs. The first is that TNCs can be expected to want to put moral responsibility for their developing-world customers ahead of the need to generate maximum profits for their developed-world stakeholders. The second belief is that TNCs have gained so much power since around 1960 that it is impossible to regulate them externally. To this author, the first belief seems incredibly naive and the second a counsel of despair. If we are to achieve the MDGs, as I argued in Chapter 1, the UN and its agencies will have to be able to exercise transnational power much more effectively than they can at present.

As indicated above, the UN has tried with regard to breast-milk substitutes. They drew up a Code under the aegis of the WHO and UNICEF, and their effort constitutes one of the most protracted attempts to achieve international control of an industrial sector. However, Nestlé and other TNCs engaged in similar production have strongly resisted anything but self-regulation with regard to the Code – officially referred to as the International Code of Marketing of Breast-Milk Substitutes, or 'the Code' for short. It has been in operation since 1981.

How TNCs try to interfere with implementation of the Code

Now, 25 years on, the advertising of breast-milk substitutes has become less blatant, as the companies involved struggle to maintain their grip. For instance, most such products now state on their packaging that breastfeeding is generally superior. In addition, many of the TNCs concerned maintain that they fully support the Code. For example, Nestlé stated as early as 1998 that it has:

> Actively encouraged national adoption of the WHO Code, with strict measures backed up by impartial and effective monitoring. ... Nestlé strictly adheres to national codes and all relevant legislation.[12]

However, international and local monitoring carried out by various NGOs and other groups shows that Nestlé and other TNCs continue to violate the Code. The strictures imposed by the Code have been explained in detail previously by this author.[11] They include restrictions on the use of the media to promote the product, and not supplying maternity wards with free starter kits, yet these restrictions are still being contravened, and such violations are on the increase.[13] It is left to national governments in poor countries to police the Code. This is rather cynical, as the TNCs can divert large sums of money and powerful forces to render such efforts futile. In fact, a number of the TNCs involved, including Nestlé, have published their own interpretations of the Code in such a way as to allow prohibited strategies to continue. In 1982, Dr A Tarutia from Papua New Guinea advised the WHO that Nestlé's activities in this context constituted an offence.[14]

Threats of trade retaliation

In 1997, Zimbabwe was on the verge of passing a law in support of the Code, and Nestlé threatened to withdraw from the country. The proposed legislation, it was estimated, would involve about 200 job loses and a serious loss of farmers supplying the milk. All of the TNCs involved lobbied the Zimbabwean government. They argued that the proposed legislation was contrary to economic growth and the development of trade liberalisation and foreign investment. However, Zimbabwe remained firm and passed the legislation. Nestlé still operates there.

TNCs have also attempted to undermine the Code by claiming that it interferes with 'freedom of commercial speech.' In South Africa, the infant food industry formed a well-endowed agency called the 'Freedom of Commercial Speech Trust.' This body then claimed that implementing the Code would jeopardise the role that commercial advertising plays in informing HIV-positive mothers about how bottle feeding can prevent transmission of the virus! In Swaziland, the infant food industry used a similar strategy. In that case, the government listened to the arguments put forward by the companies and called a representative of the International Baby Food Action Network (IBFAN) in Africa to comment on them. It then weighed up both inputs and ended up requesting the companies 'not to educate the public about HIV and breastfeeding, as that was the government's responsibility.'[15]

This brings into focus the legislative difficulties involved in likening a corporation to a virtual person, because 'freedom of speech' – whether it be 'commercial' or otherwise – is a fundamental human right under the UN Charter. However, there is no 'corporate' right to the free flow of commercial communication.

The infant food industry has been extremely resourceful in finding ways to combat the Code's legitimacy. In Pakistan, Nestlé wrote a letter to the country's Ministry of Health in which it described the proposed pro-Code legislation as 'impractical' and lacking support from paediatric consultants as well as from the industry. This attempt was stymied when the Paediatric Association voted for the Code. In India, the industry actually tried to challenge the legitimacy of the Code in the courts in 1992. This attempt also failed. Nestlé has worked assiduously to be recognised as a 'responsible citizen' that only wants to help by being involved in monitoring the Code – but this, of course, would be rather like hiring a fox to guard the chicken coop! The infant food industry as a whole has also been active in such lobbying in Pakistan, Sri Lanka, Swaziland, Zimbabwe and Gabon, among other countries.

In 1998, Nestlé complained to the Ministry of Health that it had not been invited to participate in the drafting of the national law, and even reprimanded the drafting body for its 'apparent lack of desire for dialogue!'[16] In 1996, delegates of the World Health Organization, anticipating such strategies on the part of the TNCs, urged all of its member states to ensure that monitoring of the application of the Code was transparent, independent and free from commercial influence.[17]

Self-regulation: obstacle to human rights

In the author's view, all of the above clearly illustrates that self-regulation by such corporations is ineffective. Neoliberal apologists, of course, argue that unfettered markets deliver goods and services more efficiently and should therefore be left alone, and that the public welfare is best served by letting market forces resolve the issues. However, this argument assumes that the free market itself is unregulated. Obviously this is not the case, and almost never was. The real question should be 'What type of regulation allows markets to compete as efficiently as possible while being prevented from allowing such competition to harm consumers?' This has been recognised as valid within industrial countries since the twentieth century. It is just that now we must do it internationally.

However, bodies like the WTO are implacably opposed to such an idea, and even do their best to prevent individual nations from passing such protective legislation within their own country. Countless practices of TNCs thus remain beyond legislative control. Harris Gluckman and Riva Krut argue persuasively that:

> It is as important to put regulations in place internationally as it is [to do so] nationally. A systematic method to regulate and set minimum standards for international business activity is crucial to the achievement of some critical elements of international social life and development.[18]

The United Nations Research Institute for Social Development (UNRISD) endorses this view that the 'market' will not act as some kind of invisible hand for ultimate social good. As they say:

> Left to their own devices, TNCs are likely to fulfil their responsibility in a minimalist and fragmented fashion. Their strategies may be conducive to economic growth and the stability of their operating environments, but not necessarily to sustainable human development. They still need strong and effective regulation and a coherent response from civil society.[19]

The issues raised by TNCs striving to avoid any kind of external control are of crucial importance to the whole thrust and aims of this book – hence the emphasis that this author is placing on the strategies and details. The TNCs are not giving up easily, and their malign impact in promoting malnourishment of infants and children in the LDCs needs to be opposed. They have also exerted pressure on two other fronts, namely public relations (PR) and 'dialogue', which we need to consider briefly.

Public relations and dialogue: your friendly local TNC

As part of a protracted campaign, the TNCs that promote breast-milk substitutes and other 'baby foods' have, in an attempt to deflect criticism, turned in a big way to both PR campaigns and that very cosy concept of 'dialogue.' PR has long been a concealed instrument of corporate power, and includes encouraging scientists to make statements which can be used to support corporate intent, sponsoring 'conferences' and even scholarships for such people, and so on. They expend tremendous energy on research designed to access the socio-political environment in which their companies operate, keeping 'unsavoury' issues out of public debate, delaying potentially hostile legislation, and developing a 'friendly' face in children's groups. The latter approach has included sponsoring fairs and other child-friendly activities which also attract media coverage.

At the more sophisticated end of the spectrum, 'partnerships' are promoted with NGOs and individuals active in working with children. In all of this, the public and NGOs are encouraged to work with the corporation, instead of stirring up controversy. The aim is to establish a spirit of 'We are all in this together, trying to do the best for our children, because after all what is good for the children is good for us!' Those people who continue to shout warnings and to oppose them can then be marginalised as 'misguided' or naive academics 'who aren't working to face reality.'

Even when such strategies fail to persuade the more astute non-government agencies, governments often fall for them by acting in acquiescence with WTO policies.

Government regulation linked to PR and dialogue

Attempts to foster a cosier relationship between TNCs, local people and international opinion do not only involve baby food. Indeed, at all levels of institutionalising the violation of human rights in the less developed world, TNCs and other financial agencies play a pivotal role. Governments of the USA, the UK and Germany have entered into partnership with the private sector since as far back as 1994. The governments concerned, using their own PR, try to persuade us that this is most beneficial for LDCs relying on their aid.[20] These governments even cooperate with private firms' advertising, and count it as some kind of 'social audit.' In addition to this, a number of TNCs try to involve local NGOs (which are invariably short of resources for their work), and the UN itself, in their promotional campaigns.[21] As a result, there has been a sharp increase in 'partnerships' between private firms and such agencies as the UN Conference on Trade and Development (UNCTAD) and the World Health Organization.[22]

For instance, at the 1999 World Economic Forum,[23] UN Secretary General Kofi Annan proposed a 'Global Compact' of 'shared values and principles ... in the area of human rights, labour conditions and environmental protection.' In exchange for UN support of free trade, Kofi Annan asked member companies of the International Chamber of Commerce (ICC) to 'make sure that in your own corporative practices you do not become complicit in human rights abuse.' The ICC, by the way, is a business association of over 7,000 TNCs from 130 countries.[24] Are we beginning to see the privatisation of the UN?

In the final chapter of this book, I shall describe some of the ways in which the UN will have to change if it is to fulfil its Charter aims on human rights. However, if it were to fall under the spell of neoliberalism itself, alternative approaches to transnational mediation of global equity would have to be considered.

Child slavery

The very word 'slavery' is objectionable, especially (and for good historical reasons) in Africa. Even UNICEF, that paramount advocate of children's rights, avoids using the word in the context of violation of human rights. However, slavery, defined by the *Oxford English Dictionary* as 'bondage to a master or household as a slave', is exactly what we are describing as the fate of numbers of children.[25]

The same source defines a slave as 'one who is legally bound in absolute obedience and servitude to a person or household to perform labour.'[25]

Around 200,000 children a year are sold into slavery in Africa.[26] The BBC World Service, which broadcast this figure, did so in the context of news reports about a ship bearing slave children having become lost at sea and rescued off the west coast of Africa. Hundreds of children were feared dead, and aid agencies warned that they might have been thrown overboard in order to avoid prosecution of the boat runners. If that were so, it would not be the first time. Thus, when the ship *Etireno* was finally escorted into Cotonou Port in Benin at 2am on 17 April 2001, the world's press was waiting.

Only 23 children were found on board. The adults with them all evaded contact with either the press or the authorities. Who were the children and how did they become commodities in the flourishing slave trade?

Children of the Etireno

All of the children were under 14 years of age, and most of them were under 10. They were taken into the care of a Swiss charity, 'Terre Des Hommes', where their stories gradually emerged. The BBC broadcast, which lasted for 30 minutes, was replete with specific detail because the children were very articulate and could speak clearly. They said that strangers had come to their village, paid money to their fathers and then taken them away to work in other countries. Victoire, aged 9 years, stated: 'The man's name was Jean. He gave my father [US equivalent of 75 cents] and the same amount to my brothers to share.' Another child, 6-year-old Adakoun, had been afraid to go, but her mother insisted: 'My mother told me that my father would be sad and that we would all die of starvation. So I agreed.'

The children had been at sea for nine days, when they were forced to climb overboard and hide in small boats. However, soldiers caught them and they were beaten and attacked by dogs. They were then put back on the ship and drifted for days as supplies ran out: 'On the boat we were told that if we did not stop crying, they would throw us out.'

After a few days of tender care, they gradually resumed their childhood again, as the authorities tried to reunite them with their parents. Thankfully, they were unaware of what would have happened to them if they had reached their intended destination of Gabon, where there is a lucrative trade in child slaves. Even children as young as 5 years work as housemaids, often under brutal conditions. Their names are changed and they are forbidden to speak in their own language.

They tend to get sold over and over again, and when they are too old to work as child slaves, they are thrown out on to the streets to survive on their own. The roots of this trade extend far back in West African history, and were already well established locally long before the Europeans became involved in the slave trade. In West Africa, a poor child is often sent away – possibly even abroad – to live with a wealthy relative, there to be given a better chance in life. In exchange, the child does a little work around the house. Today, however, this practice has become a business. Traffickers will buy a child for around US$ 15.00 and sell him or her for US$ 300.00 in Gabon. Philomene, who was formerly involved as an intermediary in this terrible trade, is now retired, but she described how for nine years she regularly took such children to Nigeria to sell them.

> We used to take about 80 or 100 children a year. Why? Because their
> parents give birth but don't have the money to look after children. So
> we would tell them that influential people in Nigeria are looking for
> children and that they will be treated well.[26]

She then chuckled and said that this, of course, was a lie.

Slavery in West African history

West Africa bore the brunt of the European slave trade in Africa, and hence local
people do not want to hear what has been described above referred to as 'slavery.' The Benin Government has (finally) admitted that the *Etireno* was involved
in the trafficking of children, but insists that this did not involve slavery!

Why does even UNICEF avoid using the word 'slavery' to describe what is happening? The reasons are political but not difficult to work out. Benin, and West
Africa generally, was the main focus in the worldwide trade of seventeenth- and
eighteenth-century slavery, without which neither the great sugar estates in the
West Indies, nor the cotton fields of the Deep South in the USA, nor even the
prosperity of many eminent people in Bristol could have been sustained. The idea
of slavery, even on a less vast scale, still being alive and well in West Africa is
highly distasteful to the local political leaders. For UN agencies and others to be
able to work effectively anywhere, they cannot afford to offend the sensitivities
of the local political establishments.

Readers in the UK will recall the case of Victoria Climbié, who at 8 years of age
finally died of cruelty and neglect at the hands of a distant relative of her mother.
Under an arrangement common in many African cultures, Victoria travelled from
her home to London with a woman barely known to her mother but who presented herself as a 'great aunt'. She promised that Victoria would be given the
advantages of a good British education, etc. There she suffered unspeakably cruel
treatment and subsequently died.

The trafficking of child slaves continues, often by the most modern of means.
The BBC broadcast from which most of this information is derived goes on to
describe how the reporters secretly filmed a child-slave trafficker on an Air
Gabon flight, as he was taking three children to another destination. Again, of
course, poverty lies at the root of the situation, with parents who are unable to
feed their children being easily persuaded to part with them.

The Benin Government is poor and that of Gabon is rich. Both are signatories
to the UN Convention on the Rights of the Child, and both countries have had
democratic governments for at least a decade. However, neither country has
agreed to ban this overt practice of child slavery or to punish the traffickers. Of
course, such legislation could be used by the IMF as conditionality for loans, but
it is not in the interests of such agencies to interfere in international business,
especially with Gabon.

Child sexual exploitation

This most grievous form of child exploitation is growing by leaps and bounds,
very much expedited on the one hand by more sophisticated methods of using
computers and on the other by growing disparities in wealth both within and
between countries. It is a scourge that affects both rich and poor nations, but the

main focus in this necessarily brief discussion of this crime will be in the context of financial exploitation of LDCs by the developed world. Some of these issues have already been addressed in Chapter 8.

It is known that about two million children are commercially exploited for sex each year, at least 500,000 of them in the developed nations, but some of these have been trafficked from poorer countries. The trafficking and sale of people generally is now the third largest organised crime industry (the sale of arms being the largest, and that of addictive drugs being the second largest).[27]

The sexual exploitation of children is global, but is most prevalent in countries that are beset by poverty, political upheaval and corruption. For instance, it thrives in Cambodia, where the prostitution of girls as young as 5 years is common, as many 'sex tourists', primarily from the developed countries, visit Cambodia with the specific aim of sexually abusing very young girls. Of course such individuals often do not have to travel in order to indulge their perversions, as many young girls are trafficked in the USA and the EU countries for this purpose.

One of the many factors that increase the risk of commercial sexual exploitation of a child is the extreme poverty that forces their family to sell them. Children naturally suffer severe physical and psychological problems as a result of being exploited in this way. The younger they are, the more likely they are to contract a number of sexually transmitted diseases, including HIV/AIDS. A large proportion of children who are forced into the sex trade are also dependent on various narcotic drugs.[28]

As was indicated previously, neoliberal globalisation of finance has had a major effect in indirectly increasing the incidence of child sexual exploitation. Various instrumentalities that support such globalisation, like the WTO, encourage poor countries to rely more heavily on the tourist trade. In such situations, women and children are more vulnerable to becoming commodities. Pino Arlaccki, who heads up UN efforts to curb globalised crime, has gone on record as saying that 'slavery is one of the most undesirable consequences of globalisation.'[29]

Like other forms of globalisation, the Internet is almost free of any regulation. Its international outreach means that local or national laws or customs in most LDCs are rendered ineffective. However, it is worth noting that the same technology will almost certainly play a crucial role in curbing the excesses of neoliberal economic policies and of computer abuse. The author says this having personally seen the hugely empowering impact on communities in the less developed world of gaining access to computers and their associated technology. As will be discussed in Chapter 10, giving children themselves access to a wide education, through exposure to radio, TV and computers, will no doubt play a leading role in helping them to confront sexual abuse by being more able to assert themselves.

Sexual exploitation in the context of disasters

As we have seen, the problems of protecting children from sexual abuse and exploitation are legion, but large-scale disasters raise extra problems in this regard. I am using the term 'disasters' to refer to both man-made and natural upheavals that completely – and usually suddenly – disrupt normal civil society. Such events produce huge numbers of refugees, leading to children finding themselves unaccompanied and separated from their usual surroundings. Of course even slow-onset disasters (such as drought leading to famine) can have exactly the same consequences so far as the vulnerability of children to exploitation is concerned.

Even when children, in the aftermath of a disaster, appear to be less vulnerable because they are with their parents (or other adults), they may in fact be extremely vulnerable because of pressures on their carers. Whatever the context, it is important to appreciate that a legal and policy framework already exists under UN mandate to protect vulnerable children. The UN Convention on the Rights of the Child, along with its various additional protocols, clearly delineates the child's rights. For instance, all refugees, including children, are supposed to be protected by the UN High Commission for Refugees (UNHCR). And even if people have not actually crossed borders (and therefore are not refugees), they are classed as *internally displaced persons (IDPs)*, and can still claim the protection of the UNHCR.[30]

However, disasters generate unequal power relations, from which abuse almost invariably arises. As has already been noted, the UN itself has recently come under widespread media attack in the USA with claims of sexual abuse of children in refugee camps in various parts of the world by 'UN staff.' Some of this reportage has been directed at Kofi Annan's leadership, but care is required here. Neither Kofi Annan nor the UN officials in New York and Geneva personally appoint most UN staff in disaster zones. Such staff are appointed locally and are not necessarily committed to the moral goals of the UN itself.

For instance, the UN peace-keeping mission in the Democratic Republic of the Congo confirmed that this problem was widespread.[31] In that context, 'UN staff' were accused of bartering food and small sums of money with girls as young as 13 years. The same kind of thing happens with NGOs. A refugee child in Liberia was quoted as follows:

> When Ma asked me to go to the stream to wash plates, a peacekeeper asked me to take off my clothes so that he could take a picture. When I asked him to give me money he told me, no money for children, only biscuit.[32]

And a similar quote from the same source:

> It is difficult to escape the trap of the NGO people; they use the food as bait to get you to have sex with them.[33]

An important aspect of ensuring the effectiveness of transnational mediation of human rights, as discussed in the final chapter of this book, is that a universal code of conduct for all humanitarian workers and peace-keepers be formerly implemented. As Stephanie Delaney points out in the cited article:

> Training in codes of conduct is required, both of the humanitarian workers themselves and of the affected communities. Such codes need to be given authority by enforcement and by the existence of established channels of complaint. This is vitally important because abuse of power can occur anywhere up the chain of command.[30]

The importance of this cannot be overstated. Desperate situations, such as the 2005 Tsunami, call for desperate resources, and thousands of well-intentioned people from more fortunate areas of the world feel impelled not only to give money or materials, but to throw themselves into the aid effort. However, caution is needed, and this would be facilitated by the existence of an internationally accepted Code. A particularly ghastly example of the kind of thing to which the author is referring was a report in *The Australian* newspaper that 20 Australian paedophiles attempted to travel to Indonesia and Thailand after the Tsunami, and were only apprehended because their names came up on a child offender register.[33]

Other specific issues

All of the above has by no means exhausted the topic of systematic violation of children's rights under the Charter. For instance, the author has not mentioned such phenomena as the use of children in war, child labour and the haunting incidence of child-headed households. All of these atrocities are, either directly or at least indirectly, a source of increased profit on the part of some developed-world agencies. For instance, much of the reluctance to approve a UN-brokered peace in Sudan and Darfur stems from the fact that there are powerful US and EU interests which are anxious to gain preferential access to Sudan's' oil, sexual abuse of children and the use of child soldiers not withstanding. Likewise, sweatshop child labour in unsafe factories for 10 to 12 hours a day in many parts of Asia – and elsewhere – is not something that many First World interests want to examine too closely. The shoes, clothing, etc., that are produced are just too profitable.

The most effective guarantors of children's rights are children themselves. However, only if they can get their hands on the levers of their own enhancement can we make progress in this direction. The first step is to make sure that – at the very least – every child who possibly can be is taught to be literate in their own language. Literacy is basic to all other forms of education or schooling, and is the single most important stepping-stone to self-actualisation and community advocacy.

References

1 UN Convention on the Rights of the Child, Brussels; www.unicef.org/crc/ (accessed 26 June 2006).
2 UNICEF. *A Framework for the Protection, Care and Support of Orphans and Vulnerable Children Living in a World with HIV/AIDS*; www.aidsalliance.org/sw492.asp (accessed 16 May 2006).
3 Oxfam. *The Cost of Childbirth: how women are paying the price for broken promises on aid;* http://oxfam.org.uk/what_we_do/issues/debt_aid/bp52_childbirth (accessed 16 May 2006).
4 Farmer R, Miller D. *Lecture Notes on Epidemiology and Public Health Medicine.* 3rd ed. Oxford: Blackwell; 1997. pp. 77–80.
5 Oxfam, op. cit., p. 1.
6 BBC World Service. *Children's Rights.* Broadcast on 10 May 2006; www.bbc.co.uk/worldservice/people/features/childrensrights (accessed 11 May 2006).
7 Save the Children. *State of the World's Mothers;* www.savethechildren.org/publications/sown_2006_final.pdf (accessed 11 May 2006.
8 Oxfam, op. cit., p. 4.
9 Oxfam, op. cit., p. 17.
10 Save the Children. *Global Infant Mortality Rates (2006).* www.GlobalHealthFacts.Org (accessed 11 November 2006).

11 MacDonald T. *Health, Trade and Human Rights.* Oxford: Radcliffe Publishing; 2006. pp. 61–81.

12 Nestlé. *Nestlé: complying with the WHO Code.* Yevey, Switzerland: Nestlé; 1998. p. 6.

13 *Companies Violate the 25-year-old Marketing Code.* 21 May 2006. www.ibfan.org/site2006/Page/article.php?art_id=420.

14 International Forest Marketing. *Briefing document*; www.globalwitness.org/projects (accessed 11 November 2006).

15 Richter J. *Engineering of Consent: uncovering corporate PR.* Corner House Briefing Paper No. 6. Penang, Malaysia: International Baby Food Action Network; 1998. p. 11.

16 Richter J. *Engineering of Consent: uncovering corporate PR.* Corner House Briefing Paper No. 20. Penang, Malaysia: International Baby Food Action Network; 1998. p. 7.

17 International Baby Food Action Network; www.babymilkaction.org (accessed 17 May 2006).

18 Gluckman H, Krut R. *Everything For Sale.* Chicago: University of Chicago Press; 1999.

19 United Nations Research Institute for Social Development (UNRISD). *Visible Hands: taking responsibility for social development.* Geneva: UNRISD; 2000.

20 For a Critique of World Bank 'dialogues', see www.developmentgap.org and www.irn.org. An October 2001 *Financial Times* guide to 'responsible business' suggests that the majority of initiatives to encourage corporate responsibility should not be a matter of legislation, but should instead 'be developed and overseen by new social partnerships and corporate codes of conduct, with companies seeking to "reduce risk by linking their codes to partnerships that involve human rights and development NGOs."' See Pike A. Introduction. In: *Responsible Business in the Global Economy: a* Financial Times *Guide.* October 2001, p. 5.

21 Frankel C. One foot in the future. *Tomorrow.* 1999; **9:** 11. Cited in Utting P. *Business Responsibility for Sustainable Development.* Geneva: United Nations Research Institute for Social Development; 2000.

22 Several UN agencies have turned to commercial sources of funding partly because their funding from governments has declined.

23 The World Economic Forum describes itself as 'the leading interface for global business/government interaction.' It aims to create 'partnerships between and among businesses, political, intellectual and other leaders of society to define, discuss and advance key issues on the global agenda.' See www.weforum.org (accessed 14 December 2001).

24 'UN Secretary General proposes Global Compact on Human Rights, Labour, Environment' (press release, 1 February 1999); www.un/org/partners/business/davos/htm (accessed 17 January 2001).

25 Murray J (ed.) *Oxford English Dictionary.* Oxford: Oxford University Press; June 2006.

26 BBC World News. *The Slave Children.* Broadcast on 5 October 2001.

27 Youth Action Program International. *Commercial Sexual Exploitation of Children and Child Trafficking.* p. 1; www.yapi.org/csec/ (accessed 17 May 2006).

28 Youth Action Program International, op. cit., p. 2.

29 Hughes D. *Globalising the Sexual Exploitation of Women and Children.* Coalition Against Trafficking in Women; http://action.web.ca/home/catw/readingroom.shtml?x=16747 (accessed 17 May 2006).

30 Delaney S. *Protecting Children From Sexual Exploitation in Disasters and Emergency Situations.* Bangkok: ECPAT International; 2006. p. 26.

31 UN Secretary General. *Report on Children and Armed Conflict*; www.redbarnet.dk/default.asp?ID=4468 (accessed 17 May 2006).

32 Delaney S, op. cit., p. 39.

33 Delaney S, op. cit., p. 35.

Chapter 10

Literacy and education

Primary education and literacy

The second Millennium Development Goal (MDG 2) calls for universal primary education. This is a fundamental basis for any civil society in which human rights are to be respected. However, its effect is long term in that it is applied to young children, and such people do not generally become significantly important in determining their society's direction until at least a decade, usually more, after they have commenced primary schooling. And, as the reader will be quick to realise, it is primary education's conferral of literacy, more than any other skill, that renders it so crucial. A broadly literate adult population is pivotal in sustaining the necessary levels of analysis and debate for human rights to flourish.

Having had the privilege of serving in many less developed societies, in both education and health, this author has often had occasion to note the almost immediate impact of literacy on people's awareness of their health rights, and then their organising the most effective ways of realising those rights. Hence, alongside the establishment of universal primary education, a well-resourced campaign to eradicate adult illiteracy needs to be pursued. Widespread adult illiteracy characterises the overwhelming majority of less developed societies. Indeed, it is the degree to which they can overthrow that yoke that will determine their social liberation and movement towards real development.

Therefore, before considering primary education generally, the author proposes to deal with the issue of what he calls 'institutional' adult illiteracy – that is, a situation in which a significant proportion of the adult population has traditionally been illiterate and has accepted that situation as 'natural.' Such people are easily exploited within their own country, and the country as a whole takes on characteristics that keep it underdeveloped and prey to exploitation by developed-world financial interests. The proof of this claim lies in the hostility with which developed-world power structures react to liberation struggles and their efforts to base them on a franchise of literacy.

Literacy and autonomy

The attainment of universal access to primary education would constitute the surest long-term guarantee of achievement of global equity generally. I speak as one who has been intimately associated with literacy and whose major research focus in earlier years revolved around the cognitive and psychological context of literacy. Note at the outset that I accord 'literacy' a separate and prior place to primary education generally. It is important that the reader understands why this is so.

Most instances of widespread national illiteracy occur not only in less developed countries (LDCs), but also tend to characterise very specific types of social organisation. As Paulo Freire[1] pointed out in the late 1950s, poor and especially agrarian societies tend to consist largely of two classes of people – the elite rulers, whom

Freire calls the 'tellers', and the rest, whose role is to obey without question, and whom he calls the 'doers.' Anyone who has lived and worked in a variety of Third World countries probably recognises this scene. The two groups differ markedly from one another not only in their functions, but also in many other respects. The tellers are wealthy, can to a large degree decide what they want to do and when, and they travel easily, often abroad. They have strongly assertive personalities and they cultivate individualism and personal privacy. The doers, by contrast, are poor, have little autonomy and tend to be much more group oriented. They usually stay close to home and to where they work. Typically there are comparatively few tellers, and the great majority of the people are doers. However, the most distinctive difference between the two lies in their methods of communication within each group. The tellers write things down for one another, and in discussions they make frequent reference to books, manuals and papers. They are fully literate in at least one language, and organise their lives around written laws and regulations. The doers communicate laterally and with much emphasis on contiguity within the group. Orders and information are handed down from the tellers to the doers, and they then spread by word of mouth among the doers. The doers are usually illiterate, but not in the same sense that a non-reader in an advanced industrial society might be so classified.

When conducting his preliminary research on literacy phenomena, the author identified two distinct 'types' of illiteracy, which he termed 'incidental' and 'institutional', respectively. In developed societies, it is taken for granted that the great majority of children learn how to read and write within the first two or three years of schooling, and these skills are constantly reinforced by almost all other social activities. There are exceptions, of course, such as dyslexics or other children who fail to learn to read for various physical or psychological reasons, but these constitute a very small proportion of the total. Moreover, these few cases can generally be brought to literacy by intensive one-to-one training in synthetic phonics, even if dyslexia has been diagnosed. That is, illiteracy in highly developed First World countries can be described as 'incidental.' It is specific to the individual child and is sufficiently exceptional for such a child to be likely to be classified as having special educational needs. The illiterate child is an oddity in highly developed countries, and usually feels a sense of 'being different.' This interferes with his (about 80% of such non-readers are boys) socialisation and, if not handled sensitively, can lead to a sense of isolation and to antisocial behaviour.

Illiteracy in most less developed societies is usually 'institutional.' Of course, the incidence of dyslexia and other specifically diagnosable reading problems in such societies is probably the same as it is in developed countries. There is no reason to assume otherwise, but most children never even begin to acquire literacy in the first place. In addition, there is little felt need by the person to become literate. In the author's experience, when setting up and running adult literacy classes in various LDCs, classes would quickly fill up, but an equally rapid attrition would soon set in, especially among women who, because of their household and childcare responsibilities, could have benefited most from becoming literate.

However, as the author quickly discovered, if an adult in an illiterate community did become literate, he or she often felt increasingly excluded by his or her friends and family, whose suspicions were aroused by their colleague's newly acquired skill as he or she began to process information differently and became more and more like a 'teller.' Such people were, of course, useful to their communities because of their ability to read and to apprehend argument and instruction. Characteristically, then, they became rather like non-commissioned officers in the army – not entirely trusted by the troops, but not welcomed by the officer class either![2]

Moreover, adult women who were becoming literate were often regarded as a threat on the domestic scene by their husbands, and pressure was brought on them to drop out of their classes. Learning to read and write is immensely empowering. When literacy classes were being run in El Salvador and other Central and South American countries in the 1970s and 1980s, it was not uncommon for the programmes to be violently terminated by the landholders and the military because the classes were making the peasants 'too uppity' and more likely to question their conditions. Teaching nuns of various orders were not infrequently brutally murdered, and their bodies left on display, as a warning to people not to enrol in literacy classes.

The slower and less confrontational acquisition of literacy by young children did not generally arouse such spectacular repression, but was still not vigorously encouraged by 'doer' parents. In any case, even today, children in the LDCs often do not complete primary school because they are required to work. In the Dominican Republic in 1960, under the presidency of Rafael Trujillo, an entire year 6 class in a primary school in the capital, including their teacher, were rounded up and shot because it was found that the teacher had made critical comments to the class about the dictatorship. In 1986, the author met the only survivor of that class, who had survived because he had not attended school that day. What is significant is that, even 23 years after the event, he was still fearful and did not want his name to be used.

Before considering the primary education of children, the author is anxious that the reader should appreciate the importance of running adult literacy classes if the achievement of MDG 2 is to have any real impact.

Significance of literacy to liberation

In modern times each of the great natural liberation movements has – as least in the early stages – been undergirded by a rapid increase in adult literacy levels. Access to the printed word is politically empowering because it confers on the 'doers' much of the same information as had been used against them by the 'tellers.' The precise cognitive basis for this empowerment has been discussed by psychologists and educationalists for close to half a century, but has not yet been fully explained. Institutional illiteracy is itself not understood except that it is of obvious use to the ruling classes.

If we confine our attention for a moment to the attainment of literacy in alphabetic languages – thus ignoring Chinese and other character-based languages – we immediately note an important anomaly. The ease, or otherwise, with which adult illiterates become literate seems to have nothing to do with the degree of phonic regularity of the language concerned. For instance, English is one of the most troublesome of alphabetic languages to learn to read and write, because of its orthography. This alone means that it takes considerably longer just to learn to 'bark at the print' correctly in English than it does in, say, Spanish, Italian or

German. Yet no large society with English as its first language is characterised by high levels of illiteracy.

Spanish, on the other hand, is so straightforward in its pronunciation and orthography that the author could take any reasonably intelligent 8- or 9-year-old English-speaking children, if they were already literate in English, and teach them to read Spanish text aloud in no more than an hour. The children would not understand what they were saying, of course, but would be 'barking at the print' sufficiently accurately for any Spaniard listening to be able to understand what was being said. One certainly could not say the same for English! Yet many of the Spanish-speaking Latin American and Central American countries are characterised by high levels of adult illiteracy. Why is this so?

Cognitive processing and literacy

There are two separate sub-skills involved in reading. One is the neuromuscular, eye–brain–tongue pathway 'mastery skill' involved in turning lifeless print into spoken language by 'barking at the print' in accordance with the rules of this written language. Since the eighteenth century, many methods for inculcating this 'motor skill' aspect have been elaborated. Most of them work, after a fashion, and are very much dependent on the enthusiasm of the teacher, among other things. However, the most recent research – including that of the author – strongly indicates that the best results are consistently obtained by the strict use of synthetic phonics at the outset.[3]

What it boils down to is that people can comparatively easily acquire the 'motor skill' – rather like learning to swim or to play the piano – but that this alone does not confer the kind of 'operational literacy' that changes their lives and attitudes. What is interesting, and highly significant, is that the author's research has found that reading is one of the most 'democratic' of the skills in that, unlike most others, it is not strongly related to IQ. I have taught people with IQs as low as 60 (the average is 100) to read and write, and to be able to do so well enough to enjoy this as a pastime.[4]

Starting in 1945, as the Second World War ended, a number of countries set up national literacy campaigns to try to overcome a legacy of widespread illiteracy. This author was involved in such campaigns in Honduras, Egypt and various small South Pacific countries. Between 1945 and 1960 there were 41 such campaigns. They were all based on the 'motor skill' approach described above, teaching people to decode (read) print and to encode (write) spoken words in their native language. Moreover, they all 'worked', in that people who completed the sessions could successfully pass UNESCO-based literacy tests which they couldn't do prior to the sessions. However, over the years with subsequent testing, the percentage of literate adults gradually declined.

An outstanding exception to this was the literacy campaign initiated in Cuba between 1960 and 1961. Within a year, that campaign produced an adult literacy level of 96%, as measured by UNESCO.[5,6] Any nation scoring higher than 95% is considered by that body to be 'literate.' However, even more remarkably, subsequent UNESCO measures of Cuban literacy have shown that it has remained high – up to 98%, in fact, in 1978.[7] This has to be of interest to countries that are now aiming to reach the MDG target by 2015.

This author has dealt exhaustively with the highly original techniques adopted in the Cuban Literacy Campaign, and the philosophical input of the theologian Ivan Illich (in Puerto Rico) and Paulo Freire (in Brazil).[8] Its methodology has since been followed by all of the major national liberation movements.

Political and social implications of literacy

Those who wish to set up adult literacy campaigns in an LDC, in which the majority of the population has traditionally been socially and politically disadvantaged, need to be prepared for sudden and overwhelming changes to the situation.

We do not have to rely solely on the Cuban situation to appreciate this. For instance, consider the case of the former Zaire, now the Democratic Republic of the Congo. In 1960, that benighted country – which until only a short time before had been a vast backyard for Belgian and US mining interests to exploit – became free from Belgian colonial rule. A young nationalist, Patrice Lumumba, became head of the new government. He quickly made it clear that he could not be 'bought out' by developed-world mining interests that were concerned to maintain their grip on the Congo's mineral wealth.

As part of his plan of national 'rassamblement', he wanted to initiate a literacy campaign like that of Cuba. Who knows what would have happened if he had been allowed to carry it out, but in what many saw as the most blatantly cynical display of imperial greed, the resources of much of the corporate developed world were pitted against him. The media were almost unanimous in depicting him as an unspeakable villain. Stories quickly gained currency of his followers attacking Catholic mission stations, raping and murdering nuns, and so on. There was overwhelming evidence that these attacks were financed by mining corporations and carried out by mercenary groups. US government support was also evident.

Many readers may remember the rest of this sorry tale. It was said that even UN agencies were instrumental, in at least turning a blind eye, as developed-world financial interests became complicit in bankrolling Lumumba's downfall, and later that year he was captured and, while supposedly under UN protection, was tortured and murdered. His place was eventually taken by Sese Seko Mobutu, who ran the country like a personal fiefdom for 31 years. Throughout his murderous regime, in which even a casual reference to 'human rights' could land a person in jail (or worse), the USA backed him to the hilt as a 'bulwark against communism.'[9] The question has to be asked whether, if the Congo had become a self-aware, highly literate nation like Cuba in the 1960s, that large part of Africa would now be in the state of destruction and dependency that it is in today.

Universal primary education: ultimate guarantee of a literate citizenry

Of course, universal primary education (UPE) is far more expensive than adult literacy programmes, which in any case still need to keep running in the background. Not only do children need purpose-built facilities and many of them, but they also need trained teachers. This last requirement, not entirely necessary for adult literacy programmes, is extremely costly, and it takes several years at least to prepare a large enough corps of trained teachers to keep the system running. With regard to MDG 2, therefore, what progress is being made? Will the 2015 target be realised?

Unfortunately, the current indicators suggest that it will not. In 2006, the Millennium Campaign[10] provided the following stark data.

- One in four adults in the developing world – 872 million people – is illiterate. (*Source:* Oxfam UK – Education Now Campaign)
- More than 100 million children do not go to school. (*Source:* UNFPA)
- In total, 46% of girls in the world's poorest countries have no access to primary education. (*Source:* ActionAid)
- More than one in four adults cannot read or write, and two-thirds of these are women. (*Source:* ActionAid)
- Universal primary education would cost US$ 10 billion a year – that is, half of what Americans spend on ice cream. (*Source:* ActionAid)
- Young people who have completed primary education are less than half as likely to contract HIV as those who do not have an education. Universal primary education would prevent 700,000 cases of HIV each year – around 30% of all new infections in this age group. (*Source:* Oxfam)

There is almost no prospect at all that sub-Saharan African nations, as well as those in South Asia, will achieve universal primary education by 2015. Most alarming of all are the statistics relating to girls and women for, as the author has already indicated, girls who have received a primary education – and literate women – have a much greater impact on the community than do similarly educated boys and men. In addition, many countries in East Africa and Central Africa are unlikely to achieve universal primary education by the target date.

UNESCO is the most reliable source of relevant data, because it publishes a report every April, giving an account of progress made to date. The focus in 2006 was 'Literacy for Life',[11] and it is from this report that the following data were extracted.

In 2006, the *Education for All (EFA) Global Monitoring Report* stated that Burundi, Eritrea, Ethiopia, Djibouti, Kenya, Tanzania, Zambia and Zimbabwe are included on a list of 44 countries that have a low chance of achieving universal primary education by 2015. Other African countries included on that list are Benin, Burkina Faso, Chad, Egypt, Gambia, Ghana, Guinea, Ivory Coast, Madagascar, Mali, Mauritania, Mozambique and Swaziland.

However, some countries have achieved gender parity in primary and secondary education for 2005. Kenya had reached a gender ratio of 96.5% for males and 96.9% for females in primary school enrolment in 2002–03. The gross level of enrolment countrywide was 95.5%. On the other hand, Burundi, Eritrea, Rwanda, Uganda, Ethiopia, Malawi, Zimbabwe, Benin, Burkina Faso, Gambia, Mali and Mauritania are all at risk of not achieving this goal.

Of course, the Millennium Development Goals do not apply only to LDCs. Some developed countries, such as the UK and Denmark, also have a gender ratio bias, but opposite in direction to that in the less developed world. The following is a quote from the already cited 2006 report.

> In the United Kingdom, for example, the ratio of males to females enrolled in secondary education was 159.0 percent and 199.1 percent,

respectively. Similarly, in Denmark, the ratio was 125.9 percent for males and 132.4 per cent for females. Examining the literacy goal, the report shows that most countries in the East and Central African region are at serious risk of not achieving the goal. Burundi, Kenya, Rwanda and Tanzania are among the 30 countries that are at serious risk of not achieving the goal of adult literacy by 2015. Thirty countries are at serious risk of not achieving the goal by 2015 because their very low literacy rates are not increasing fast enough. Most of these countries are in Africa, but the list also included India, Nepal and Pakistan, and several Latin American countries.[11]

However, it should be noted that performance does not depend on percentage of gross domestic product (GDP) devoted to education. Expenditure on education in developed countries, such as Canada, the USA and the EU countries, rarely reaches even 15%, but in more than half of the countries in sub-Saharan Africa it exceeds this level. More than 25% of the GDP of the budgets of Botswana, Guinea, Mexico and Morocco is devoted to educational spending.[12] Kenya, Uganda and Tanzania are highlighted in the UNESCO report because they have abolished primary school fees altogether, as have Zambia and Cape Verde. Although it is true that a number of countries have increased their educational spending, there has been considerable duplication and wastage. There is also evidence of inadequate auditing and misappropriation in the most needy communities, in a sense financing the more affluent in society at the expense of the poor.

It is also clear from the report that there are many factors that impede the attempts of poor countries to institute a policy of Education for All (EFA), including poorly trained teachers, huge enrolments that compromise quality, hostile learning environments (especially for girls), and levels of poverty that we can barely comprehend. This author has often visited classrooms in Papua New Guinea, Mozambique, Burundi and elsewhere, in which more than 80 children are crammed together in stifling heat and sun – with only one portable, badly scratched blackboard.

Such schools often also lack indoor plumbing, and the facilities that are available are shared by both sexes. A frequent distraction, too, even if the children are quiet, is caused by noisy adjacent classrooms, insects buzzing about in the heat, and so on. Teaching under such conditions is exhausting.

The need to go beyond MDG 2

Universal primary education is certainly a necessary basis for guaranteeing literacy in society generally, but if it stops there, disruptions to the economy soon make themselves manifest. Low-level work cannot be found for all of those who have graduated from primary school. At the same time, those who will run the country (Civil Servants, teachers, medical staff, etc.) must ultimately be trained 'at home', otherwise the country will always be largely run by foreign personnel.

As things stand now in sub-Saharan Africa, for instance, less than one-third of young people receive any secondary education, and fewer than half of those who start it ever complete it. Sub-Saharan African countries are struggling to achieve universal primary education, but before achieving that, they need to urgently elaborate strategies for widening the base for secondary education.

The country's economic and social development, and the people's very dignity, rely on it. These needs are not lost on developed-world financial institutions like those of Bretton Woods. It is in the interest of any effective imperial power to be able to run their colonies – at the middle-management level – by training recruits from the colony itself.

Typically, the British Empire was reasonably adept at training up corps of indigenous people to 'run the shop' for them, and it was those people who tended to take over as leaders when the countries gained their independence. Other European colonial powers did not do as effective a job, and thus the independence of those countries raised many more problems. The author was made painfully aware of this when he was privileged to have an interview with Patrice Lumumba two weeks after he gained power in the former Belgian Congo. As Lumumba pointed out, independence would prove very difficult for the Congo because the cadres of locally trained Congolese were just too small. Lumumba himself had only been formally educated by the Belgians as a post office clerk, but he had set about educating himself in his spare time.

At present things are not being left to chance in this way in the LDCs. The World Bank has developed a study to prepare post primary training programmes in sub-Saharan Africa in order to train local personnel to manage the economies of their countries. This study is called Secondary Education in Africa (SEIA). It is financed by the World Bank, along with various international donors and other African countries. European contributing bodies include the Norwegian Education Trust Fund, the Irish Trust Fund, the Dutch Trust Fund and the French government. The eventual total cost of the SEIA study is estimated to be nearly US$ 2 billion.[13]

The objectives of the study are as follows:

- to support sub-Saharan African countries in developing strategic agendas for secondary education reforms
- to collect and summarise best practices and identify sustainable development plans for expanding and improving the quality, equity and efficiency of junior and senior secondary education in sub-Saharan Africa, and to disseminate information through workshops and conferences
- to find ways for donor agencies to better coordinate and support the SEIA reform agenda.

The study was set up in 2002, and has now almost completed most of the background work.

This is a wonderful initiative for the countries concerned – or it could be. Whether it is or not will depend on the extent to which, once the infrastructure is established, it comes under local control. Those countries desperately need to develop, if global equity is to be realised, and it is important that they are linked into the global trading framework. For all of this to redound to the strengthening of global human rights, great care will have to be taken and considerable wisdom exercised. More will be said about this in the final chapter of this book.

References

1 Freire P. *Pedagogy of the Oppressed*. San Francisco, CA: Seabury Press; 1974. pp. 78–81.
2 MacDonald T. The two illiteracies. In: Laura RS, MacDonald TH, editors. *Perspectives on Illiteracy*. Newcastle, NSW: University of Newcastle Press; 1984. pp. 9–32.

3 House of Commons. *Teaching Children to Read. Education and Skills Committee, Eighth Report of Session 2004–05.* London: The Stationery Office; 2005. pp. 66–80.

4 MacDonald T. *The Road to Reading.* London: Aurum Press; 1998. p. 6.

5 Lorenza A. *Report on Methods and Means Utilized in Cuba to Eliminate Illiteracy.* Paris: UNESCO; 1969. pp. 22–37.

6 Fagan R. *The Transformation of Political Culture in Cuba.* Stanford, CA: Stanford University Press; 1969. p. 51.

7 Kozol J. A new look at the literacy campaigns in Cuba. *Harvard Educ Rev.* 1978; **48:** 341–77.

8 Illich I. *After De-Schooling – What?* London: Writers and Readers Press; 1973. pp. 10–12.

9 Patrice Lumumba's replacement by Moise Tshombe was widely regarded at the time. A full account can be found at www.reelingreviews.com/lumemba.htm

10 Millennium Campaign. *Voices Against Poverty. Goal 2. Achieve universal primary education;* www.millenniumcampaign.org/site/pp.asp?c=grKVL2NLE (accessed 6 June 2006).

11 Nkinyangi S. *Literacy for Life.* Nairobi: UNESCO Nairobi Office; 2006. pp. 2–40.

12 Millennium Campaign, op. cit., p. 31.

13 World Bank. *Secondary Education in Africa;* www.worldbank.org/afr/seia (accessed 6 June 2006).

Chapter 11

Impact of the globalisation of HIV/AIDS

Naught for our comfort

In 2005 the media became very much preoccupied with the possibility that avian flu would become pandemic, with people infecting one another directly. This gave rise to alarming headlines, books and films, and people all over the world have been terrified by the prospect. But why spend so much energy worrying about a hypothetical pandemic when we are confronted by the real thing? HIV/AIDS is steadily destabilising communities and is now well established throughout the world – things could get very nasty, very fast. As the late Dr Lee Jong-Wook, Director General of the World Health Organization, wrote in a speech he was due to give on 22 May 2006, 'There can be no comfort level in the fight against HIV.'[1] Most tragically, Lee Jong-Wook died at the age of 61 years, while undergoing surgery for a blood clot on the brain, on the very day he was due to give that speech. As previously indicated, on 9 November 2006, Dr Margaret Chan, an equally deter-mined activist against the HIV/AIDS pandemic, was appointed Director General of WHO.

The fact is that the existing HIV/AIDS pandemic is a very real threat to all of our civilisations. However, few people seem to have realised this, for several reasons. It hasn't moved quickly, the way the Black Death did, and it has been steadily killing off millions, but mainly in the poorer countries of the world. It was first identified medically through its incidence in the USA in 1981, but we later discovered that it had been active in the African Great Lakes region for several decades, wiping out whole families and entire villages. Never mind the possibility of an avian pandemic, we were face to face with a real one!

When the disease first struck, though, leaders were slow to realise what was happening. In sub-Saharan Africa, leaders had difficulty acknowledging first of all the link between HIV and AIDS, but also its potential impact on society as a whole. More than two decades later, the message is only gradually sinking in, but now, as we shall see, the pandemic has killed millions across the globe and has left millions more socially and physically disabled. It has created generations of orphans, among whom siblings often oversee one another's slow and hideous demise. Lest we impute these facts to conditions unique to Africa, the same myopic attitudes have affected community leaders in many developed-world communities.

As Laurie Garrett[2] graphically pointed out in an article published in 2005, adequate resources for fighting HIV/AIDS have not been put in place, despite growing international political concern. As far back as 2000, the UN Security Council issued Resolution 1308, which warned that, if unchecked, the HIV/AIDS pandemic could threaten world stability and secu-rity. By 2005, AIDS had already killed nearly 30 million people, orphaning close to 15 million children and affecting in excess of 50 million people. As stated above, because so much of the more spectacular impact has been in the developing world, the widespread potential of the pandemic to cause broad social damage has been underestimated by most of the media. Its impact on child development, marriage and family relationships, agriculture and coherent political activity still does not have the media cachet of an avian flu pandemic!

However, we now know three indisputable facts about HIV/AIDS as we address the Millennium Development Goals.

1   HIV/AIDS is the most complex disease we have ever dealt with.
2   As the pandemic develops, new threats to global stability are bound to arise that interfere with such activities as global trade.
3   Research continues to suggest advances in antiretroviral treatments, but we have to make them universally available if they are to be at all effective, as Dr Chan stated in her acceptance speech.

We have faced huge pandemics before. Bubonic plague (the Black Death) has visited us several times since it made its impact felt in the fifth century BC in Greece. And, of course, there was the global flu pandemic following the First World War. However, HIV/AIDS is worse in many ways. It moves insidiously, killing its victims over a period of years, during which time they are often rejected and despised by their communities. Since 1971, it has created waves of infection, often followed years later by waves of acute disease states (there is certainly more than one terrible way to die of AIDS) in which several generations of the same family may die in the wrong chronological order. In the case of the Black Death plague in fourteenth-century Europe and of the flu pandemic in 1918–19, there were waves of infection followed later by waves of acute illness and then by deaths, sometimes of all the generations of one family, after which there was family and community breakdown.

However, with HIV/AIDS, the intervals between these waves have been as long as 14 years. The waves themselves have been staggered, with considerable variation from one person to another in the way in which the illness has manifested itself. As Garrett pointed out in his fine article, successive steep waves have passed over sub-Saharan Africa for three or four generations, while India, South-East Asia, Ukraine and Russia have been swept by shallower waves. The latter had a less immediate impact than the steeper waves in Africa, but now these areas are experiencing very high infection rates. Ahead of these waves lies the creation of generations of orphans and the large-scale breakdown of communities and of cultural values.

Before we consider these matters in more detail, let us look at the rates of infection globally at the time of writing (2006). I shall cite the UK and the USA as representing the impact of HIV/AIDS on the developed world, and the African countries, India and China as representing the impact of the pandemic on the less developed countries (LDCs). Before discussing the situation in Africa, it is important to define two words that will feature prominently in this and subsequent chapters, namely *prevalence* and *incidence*. *Prevalence* refers to the existing number of people with a given disease, either at a given time or over a given time period. *Incidence* refers to the number of new cases at a given time or over a given time period.

Africa

Since, as far as we know, the pandemic first gained a foothold in Africa, we shall start there. Right now, sub-Saharan Africa is more badly affected by HIV/AIDS than anywhere else in the world, with nearly 25 million people living with AIDS. Moreover, during 2005 about 2.7 million new infections occurred, and during that time at least 2 million people died in this region. And in sub-Saharan Africa more than 12 million children have already been orphaned by HIV/AIDS.

The link with education is multidimensional. On the one hand, there is the need for people to understand the infection and how it is spread. These matters can and should be dealt with in schools to which all young people have access – and as early as possible. Until recently, for instance, even among people who agreed that public schools should provide sex education, the belief was widely held that this should not start until the secondary level. However, countries that have records available on sex education, such as Cuba, long ago realised that postponing such education until secondary school is leaving it far too late. As the author has described previously,[3] even in the 1970s, Cuban children as young as 8 or 9 years of age were being taught the full details, to the extent (in one class that I witnessed) of having them examine human fetuses in the lab and discuss the implications of childbirth, marriage, and so on.

However, links with education have to extend all the way up the educational ladder if they are to have an optimal impact on regressive and discriminatory cultural practices. In Chapter 8, allusion was made to the practice of lobola. The evils of that system can only be addressed by community education for women in particular. However, between 1989 and 1999, Zimbabwe reduced spending on such educational programmes by almost 50%.[4] It goes without saying that HIV prevention strategies, which should ideally be discussed in such contexts, have been even further affected by spending cuts in the last five years.

As far back as 1990, Wilson[5] argued that his studies in sub-Saharan Africa showed that there was a high level of 'academic' knowledge about HIV transmission, but that this knowledge did not lead to appropriate sexual risk reduction practices, not even condom use! Maposphere and his colleagues[6] declared that only 38% of men in Harare reported that they used condoms. This was due to the belief, still widely held in this region, that it is harmful for a man not to satisfy his sexual urges. Furthermore, in Asian societies in general, production of offspring is considered to be almost as crucial as the virginity of the bride. Thus, whatever the health rights of the woman may dictate, condoms are often eschewed because of the belief that they represent a plot on the part of American and European interests to reduce African populations! These are just a few of the obstacles to the eradication of HIV/AIDS – obstacles that can be easily overcome by the impact of education and open discussion.

Unless there is a spectacular increase in sex education, care and treatment in Africa, it is expected that death tolls on the continent will continue to rise for the next five or six years. The implication is that the worst of the epidemic's impact is yet to come, even though its social and economic consequences are already being felt in health, education, industry, agriculture, human resources and the economy in general.[7]

Trends in the epidemic

According to WHO epidemiologists, the rate of new HIV infections in sub-Saharan Africa reached a peak in 2000 and is now levelling off (as of 2006). The term 'rate of infection' refers to the proportion of people who are infected. However, this levelling off is still taking place at a high rate of infection, auguring a very bleak future.[8]

Probably as a result of prevention campaigns, a few sub-Saharan countries have seen declines in prevalence, but elsewhere epidemics are still expanding. HIV prevalence continues to increase with population growth. Stability, of course, is reached when the death rate among those already infected equals the rate of new infections. Thus a country with a stable but very high prevalence must be experiencing a high number of AIDS deaths per year. This tends to dramatically undercut the development of entire communities. As a result, sub-Saharan Africa faces a triple challenge:

1 bringing healthcare to those who are already infected
2 providing antiretroviral drugs and other treatment, to reduce the number of new infections
3 addressing the cumulative impact of over 20 million deaths on orphans and other survivors.

Elsewhere in Africa

Other parts of Africa are affected differently. In some countries, the epidemic is still growing, and a few countries are in imminent danger of a sudden explosive growth. In Cameroon, HIV prevalence in pregnant women rose from 8% to 11% between 1998 and 2000. However, prevalence rates vary widely from country to country. Thus in Somalia and Senegal the prevalence is just below 1% of the adult population, whereas in South Africa and Zambia, around 15–20% of the adult population are infected (according to data for 2005).

Four of the sub-Saharan countries have rates of HIV infection in excess of 20%, namely Botswana (24.1%), Lesotho (23.28), Swaziland (33.4%) and Zimbabwe (20.1%). Until recently, Nigeria had a low rate, at 2% in 1993, but it had increased to 3.9% by 2005 – and Nigeria is the most populous country in Africa. In East Africa the rate exceeds 6% in Uganda, Kenya and Tanzania.[9]

Is HIV prevention feasible in Africa?

Many commentators on the HIV/AIDS scene in Africa are discouraged by the continuing rise in the rate of HIV infection. However, this must not be regarded as inevitable. This author has seen considerable evidence that prevention efforts, especially when closely linked with education, can be effective even in the most heavily infected countries. We have already mentioned Senegal, where the establishment of a vigorous AIDS education programme kept infection rates low – still only 0.9% in 2005. However, even in Uganda, where infection rates were the highest in Africa in the 1990s, these rates are now only about 5%. This is almost certainly due to the educational drive instituted by the Ugandan government in 2004. And even in Kenya and Zimbabwe, along with urban areas of Zambia and Burkina Faso, similar declines have occurred. Alongside these gains, however,

HIV infection rates have continued to increase and severe AIDS epidemics have continued to grow in South Africa, Swaziland and Mozambique.

Education is critical, of course, but without huge supplies of free condoms it will not have much impact. Along with easy access to condoms, people need to become accustomed to talking openly about sexuality, contraception, etc., and this is also linked to education. Cultural taboos seem much more resilient than they really are. When the author was a young student in French Canada, not only was information about condoms illegal, but discussion of sexual issues was regarded as 'depraved' and 'indecent.' However, in 1956, after years under a series of extremely reactionary provincial governments, Quebec suddenly elected a 'progressive' regime. Within months, ordinary press and media were discussing such previously taboo subjects as divorce, women's rights, abortion on demand, contraception, and so on. Revealing photographs of nude women, which were at first shocking, became so commonplace in theatre marquees, etc., that within a year hardly anyone batted an eye. Within the next few years, statistics on children's health, women's rights, etc. showed a sharp improvement. My home province has never looked back. The lesson is that delicacy, political correctness and an almost reverential deference to 'cultural norms' are not a way forward.

But then changes must come from the communities themselves. Importing foreign values and tastes creates its own resistances. This is why, with regard to public health issues such as AIDS, there is nothing as effective as discussion groups – backed up by good sex education programmes in primary schools.

In all of this, then, is there any place at all for developed-world involvement? Consider the statistics. In 2001, there were only 4.6 condoms per man per year in the sub-Saharan African countries. To bring the average across all of Africa up to the level of use in the six best equipped countries on the continent, we would need 19 billion more condoms. It is estimated that it would cost US$ 47.5 million a year to meet this need.[10]

Treatment provision in Africa for HIV/AIDS

We have previously referred to the sterling work of the late Director General of the WHO, Dr Lee Jong-Wook. It was he who suggested and pushed for the implementation of the famous '3 by 5' HIV/AIDS treatment programme. This programme aimed to get life-saving antiretroviral (ARV) treatment to at least 3 million victims of the pandemic by the end of 2005. Most informed public health workers argued that the campaign would fail, and indeed it did, but 1.3 million people were treated, which is itself a major achievement. However, we still have a long way to go before we can even begin to think in terms of global equity in the right to health.

UNAIDS goes on to point out that, as of 2006, fewer than 20% of the Africans who need it are receiving ARV treatment. Many more millions are not even receiving treatment for the legion of opportunistic infections to which the AIDS victim is prey. But why is this? We have come a long way with refining ARV drugs in the last decade, and in the developed world a positive result on an HIV test is no longer a death sentence, but rather an annoyingly temporary disruption to one's life.

Since 2002, we have used ARV drugs enough for biochemists to have been able to elaborate generic copies of those produced by Pfizer and other multinational pharmaceutical corporations, as discussed in Chapter 7. These generic copies can be mass produced at a much lower cost than the pharmaceutical corporations can manage, partly because the pharmaceutical corporations have had to pay out so much for the original research, and indeed five years ago both Brazil and India were among countries producing these for the Third World market. However, the pharmaceutical firms, and their backers in the US government, fought tooth and nail to halt such production and export.

In their efforts to maintain their profits, the pharmaceutical firms involved the WTO and TRIPS in order to get their way. As we shall see later in this chapter, India has caved in to the 'empire' and has outlawed those of its firms that produced such generic copies for sale outside India. This may fit in with India's needs to establish better relations with the USA, now that it is a nuclear power. However, one thing we can say is that instrumentalities like TRIPS and the WTO may be seriously impeding the fight against the pandemic. If we are to achieve even the eight Millennium Development Goals – never mind global equity in human rights generally – these impediments will have to be set aside. And indeed it appears that it has been with the WHO stated aim of achieving universal access to HIV/AIDS treatment to all who need it by 2010.

Beyond that, treatment and care for HIV/AIDS consist of elements over and above ARV drugs. These include enough food, for instance, because ARVs cannot be taken on an empty stomach. People who require ARV treatment are called upon to eat before taking the medication, maybe three or four times a day at a minimum. I personally have known of many who have had to give up ARV treatment, and leave themselves open to the ravages of AIDS, simply because they lacked the resources to feed themselves adequately. This is a disgraceful state of affairs, and in a half-decent world it would not be allowed to prevail. Other ancillary aspects necessary to give ARV treatment optimal scope include access to counselling services, regular blood tests, and treatment of other opportunistic sexually transmitted disease (STDs), as well as other infections such as tuberculosis. Malaria also readily kills off the weaker victims of AIDS.

In Africa, Botswana has pioneered the provision of ARVs. Their national treatment programme began in January 2002, and by September 2005 nearly 55,000 people were being cared for under it. According to World Health Organization figures, 85% of the people in need of ARV treatment were receiving it. Other African countries have not yet been able to follow Botswana's example, due to insufficient funds, lack of infrastructure for training the necessary corps of health workers, etc.

The way forward for Africa

Lack of finance, as stated above, is the most critical barrier to progress. However, if that problem did not exist, how would neoliberal economics work? We shall consider this problem in the last chapter. For now, suffice it to say though, money is required to set up the infrastructure to make programmes like that of Botswana universal throughout Africa. Such programmes would cover sexual and mother-to-child placental transmission of AIDS. Palliative care (pain relief), even for the dying, could be provided, opportunistic infections coped with and care for orphans implemented.

In April 2001, Kofi Annan called for the establishment of a Global Fund to Fight AIDS, Tuberculosis and Malaria. He quoted an estimate of US$ 7–10 billion being required per year to run the project, but in its first year (2001), only US$ 1.5 billion were raised by the international community. Any one of our several pointless wars far exceed US$ 10 billion a year in costs! Of that US$ 1.5 billion, Africa was given 62%, almost all of it for HIV/AIDS-related purposes.

In addition, there have been major administrative hiccups in distributing the funds. By halfway through 2003, only nine African countries had actually received any cash. But this is a worldwide pandemic that we are discussing here. Can we really presume to ask it to slow down so that governments can get their act together?

India and AIDS

This author has found that many Indians themselves have a somewhat bemused attitude to the incidence of HIV/AIDS in their own country. On the one hand, their media persuades them that they are a technologically advanced nation, with an economy sustained by successful business ventures. Surely AIDS can have no significant grip on a country that can produce its own nuclear weapons and hold commanding positions in science, the arts and businesses. In many ways it is a country still enslaved by cultural and religious practices that belong to a bygone era. On 30 June 2006, Reuters News Agency broke the news that India planned to challenge the latest UN estimates which show that it has over-taken South Africa in HIV/AIDS prevalence, and now has top place in that wretched league.

What lies behind this is that UNAIDS, the UN's AIDS watchdog, said in May 2006[11] that there were 5.7 million Indians infected, compared with 5.5 million cases in South Africa. The Indian government was quick to publicly dispute this in the media, claiming that the correct figure for India was 'only' 5.2 million cases! Of course, even that estimate bespeaks a major problem. Many Indian health pundits and academics went on record as accusing the country's govern-ment of suppressing the true figures. The Director General of India's National AIDS Control Organization, Jujatha Rao, told Reuters[12] that the discrepancy was due only to different statistical approaches, and explained this as follows:

> UNAIDS has taken a different methodology, but it has to be validated because the assumptions that UNAIDS took were based on global data and not Indian data, so they therefore came up with higher estimates.

The differences, according to Rao's further comments, arose from the fact that UNAIDS takes into account all age groups, whereas the Indian data were restricted to those aged between 15 and 49 years. Rao expects the validation process to take 6 months, which means that a useful figure for comparison will not be available until early 2007.

However, despite these objections, the figures are sufficiently worrying to have energised the Indian government to take major steps to stem the spread of the pandemic. They intend to spend the equivalent of US$ 152 million in the fiscal year 2006–07, with the bulk of this being spent on ARV treatment, the produc-tion and distribution of condoms, and media-driven educational campaigns. UNAIDS estimates that, during 2005 alone, around 400,000 HIV/AIDS-related deaths occurred. Rao has agreed that this figure is possible.

High AIDS incidence linked to human rights issues

While the Indian government has been arguing about statistics, AIDS groups in India have come to the conclusion that a major factor contributing to the country's AIDS figures has been cultural practices with regard to married women. Surveys have satisfied them that the majority of HIV-infected women had not had multiple partners, nor did they have any history of drug use or of blood transmission. Their plight had been due to their promiscuous husbands infecting them.

Reuters[13] quotes Sunitili Solomon, chairperson of the YR Gaitonde Center for AIDS Research and Education, as pointing out that investigation of these 'wronged' women means that the present research focus is inadequate and must be expanded to include married monogamous women. They may not – without being informed of current funding – realise that they are at risk because they assume that it is their own behaviour alone which determines this. They have to be educated about the social realities and helped to realise that their husbands may be putting them at risk. Solomon emphasised the point by telling the Reuters reporter:

> As more and more women become infected, notions of risk groups need to be redefined to more accurately assess the potential for HIV infections.

However, in India's deeply patriarchal society, women at present have very little say as to whether or not their husbands use condoms. The situation is changing, though, as primary education for girls becomes more common. In addition, media such as radio and email are rapidly eroding the once almost total privacy of the home environment.

Solomon's comments to the Reuters reporter were based on a study conducted by the YR Gaitonde Center for AIDS Research and Education in 2004 and 2005, which showed that 85% of a cohort of 3,357 women surveyed had had sexual relations with only one partner, namely their husband. These figures had not been considered before because previously the only groups of women to be surveyed had belonged to high-risk groups such as intravenous drug users and sex workers.

However, as implied when discussing Africa's AIDS epidemic earlier in this chapter, whatever approaches countries can adopt to prevent AIDS infection, strategies for larger-scale treatment programmes need to be elaborated, and it is here that we run into trouble with the WTO and TRIPS. Progress is being made, through pressure from the WHO itself and from pharmaceutical firms in other countries, such as India, Brazil and China, towards allowing countries to market generic copies of ARVs. This pressure has now been brought into sharp focus by the UN's 2006 stated target of access to treatment for all by 2010. To explain these recent hopeful developments, a quick rundown of the role of TRIPS and the multinational pharmaceutical corporations is necessary.

AIDS, TRIPS and generic drugs

AIDS cannot be cured, but it no longer carries the sentence of imminent death, because of the development of a sequence of ever-improving ARV treatments.

These were expensive to research and therefore costly to produce, but if it is only money standing between a victim of HIV/AIDS and a continued reasonably healthy and fulfilling life, this has to be good news – for those who can afford it. As we have seen, though, this has effectively excluded most of the most heavily infected regions in the world. However, there is some leeway, because not every country in the WTO has to observe TRIPS to the same degree. The Doha Declaration of 2000[14] made this clear especially with regard to important pharmaceuticals. Because developed countries had already had legislation on patents for a long time, they were only given one year (until 2001) to readjust their legislation for TRIPS. However, LDCs were given until 2006, and this deadline was extended to 2016 for pharmaceutical patents.

With regard to what we call 'generic copies' of ARV drugs, the reader needs to understand that there are two forms of most modern pharmaceuticals – proprietary (or brand named) and generic. Generic pharmaceuticals are either as found in nature, or very close to it (e.g. digitalis, from the foxglove plant, for certain cardiac conditions), or are copies of a proprietary drug.

Usually TRIPS rules would make it illegal to make generic copies of proprietary drugs. However, the Doha conference in 2001 issued an exemption, stating that TRIPS cannot override public health. They gave permission for countries that had not had patency laws prior to 1995 to make generic copies of pharmaceuticals patented prior to 1995. If such a country wished to copy a pharmaceutical introduced after that date, they could only do so under a system called 'compulsory licensing.' Governments can issue such licences if the pharmaceutical is unaffordable to their people. This applies only to pharmaceuticals for severe health conditions.

India, after being placed under great pressure by the WTO, finally agreed in late 2005 to prevent further production of generic copies of ARVs. To some extent, compulsory licensing laws may provide a way out. There are other countries that produce generic pharmaceuticals – the main ones being Canada, Brazil, South Africa, China and Thailand – so India is not alone. However, India is especially important because the pharmaceutical firms there produce both the finished generic tablet form of the ARV concerned and the raw ingredients and chemicals needed for its production. Many of the latter are then exported to the major TNC pharmaceuticals to enable them to produce their brand name versions.

The question then arises, under these arrangements can India be prevented from producing and marketing generic copies of ARVs? It already produces large quantities of these drugs, both for domestic use and for export. To answer this legal question, a little explanation is necessary. Only the laws of individual countries can be used to enforce the TRIPS/WTO agreements. There is not an existing international law. Suppose that X and Y were two countries such that X had no such laws on intellectual property, but Y did. In this case, a company in X could copy a product produced (under national patent) in Y. The TRIPS agreement with the WTO tries to forestall this kind of thing by encouraging member countries to build national patency laws into their legislation. If country X did so, then country Y could then register its patent with country X, and copying it would then be illegal.

In that event, India – until 2004 – was in the same position as country X. It had no regulation on product patents – only on the processes used in their manufacture, and it is for this reason that generic copy production became such a profitable industry there. So it is that, on 1 January 2005, the five-year 'grace period' given to India to help it to conform to TRIPS ended and, in October 2005, the new patent laws – to which reference has already been made – came into force.

Thus, although most of the ARVs on the WHO's list of 'essential treatments' did not become available on prescription until 1996 or later, the majority were patented in their original countries of manufacture prior to TRIPS coming into force in 1995. They can therefore continue to be produced. However, the more recent – and more effective – ARVs were patented after 1995 and before 2005, when India legislated for its TRIPS-based patent laws. The producers of these drugs – most in the highly developed countries – will file for patents in India. Such patents last for 20 years, but in that time a lot of poor people can die of AIDS! India could try to sidestep this by granting compulsory licences. However, powerful First World countries would not favour investing in a country copying its patents and underselling them to other countries in the global marketplace. India is on a neoliberal drive to 'modernise', and its actions so far seem to suggest that it is swayed more by neoliberal orthodoxy than by humanitarian principles.

What are 'modern' ARVs?

The newest ARVs are not only more effective and with fewer side-effects, but are also desperately needed as a second line of defence. When a person has been taking a certain combination of ARV drugs for some time, or has missed a few doses, their HIV can begin to mutate and become resistant to the effects of their medication. As a result, the amount of virus in their blood begins to rise, necessitating a change in their ARV regime, from first-line to second-line drugs. Proprietary first-line drugs have plenty of competition from their generic counterparts, and so can often be bought for not much more than the generic version. However, pharmaceutical companies that are producing second-line drugs have no generic competition, and can therefore charge much higher prices, which are often out of reach of people in resource-poor countries. In Cameroon, for example, the recommended first-line treatment costs US$ 277 per person per year. However, the recommended second-line treatment costs a massive US$ 4,762, because generic versions of these drugs are not widely available.[15]

The commonly used ARV drugs Truvada® (a combination of emtricitabine and tenofovir) and Aptivus® (tipranavir) are two formulations that are not currently produced generically, as they have only been patented very recently. The drugs Viread® (tenofovir) and Combivir® (a combination of lamivudine and zidovudine) are currently produced generically, but their original manufacturers are now seeking to patent them in countries such as India, as their original patent date is after 1995. If they are successful, generic manufacture would have to stop. There has been particular protest over Combivir®, as it is a very commonly used first-line treatment that combines two pre-1995 drugs (zidovudine is in fact so old, that it is now 'off' patent in many countries) which, separately, can both be copied perfectly legitimately. It is only the combined pill that has a post-1995 original patent date, and sadly this is the version most often found in developing countries.

Preparing stockpiles of second-line ARVs

China, as indicated previously, is involved in generic copying and production of ARVs, but before we move on to a consideration of China's AIDS epidemic, let us end our account of India's role and its legal situation with regard to TRIPS and the WTO. We shall attempt to anticipate what will happen with regard to the second-line defences against the global pandemic of AIDS. In attempting to 'read the runes' in this way, we should keep in mind the UN commitment to 'universal access as needed – to ARVs by 2010.' Second-line ARVs are just as important as the original ARVs because they need to be called into play when patients who are being treated with a first-line ARV develop immunity to it.

Asian countries are now very much at the top of the league in producing generic copies and a good second-line ARV defence net. Indeed, at a plenary address to the Seventh International Conference on AIDS in Asia and the Pacific (ICAAP) in Kobe, Japan, in July 2005, the WHO spokesman for UNAIDS, Jim Kim, had nothing but praise for Asia in this respect.[16] He stated that the number of people on ARVs had increased by more than 50% in the last 6 months, from 100,000 to 155,000. However, as doctors know only too well, such a rapid increase in use will generate an equally substantial rise in drug resistance and hence the need for rapid development of second-line ARVs.

Much of the less developed world now depends on Indian generic production to meet this need, but the recent revisions of Indian patent law could create an ARV access crisis and thus sabotage much of their great headway in controlling the epidemic. India's eagerness to please corporate business opinion has angered many NGOs in that country. The question arises as to whether that other restless Asian giant, China, can fill the gap. With regard to these matters, Dr Quraishi, Director General of the National AIDS Control Organisation of India, was quoted as saying:[17]

> I am very worried about the provision of second-line ARVs. We are not worried about China. Whatever produces cheap drugs is all that counts. The Indian government has played into the hands of the big international pharmaceutical corporations, and its leaders must be held accountable!

The general consensus of informal opinion seems to be that China can fill the gap. However, if China fails to do so, for whatever reasons, the implications would be bleak. All of those people who are now doing so well on generic copies of first-line ARVs will suddenly find – when immunity sets in – that they need to pay many times the price to continue treatment. This will stop the treatment of millions and surrender all of those impressive gains made against HIV/AIDS.

China's recent pronouncements do not augur well. She is eager to play by the WTO's rules. China's Vice Minister of Health, Wang Longde, said at the ICAAP meeting referred to above that 'when China joined the WTO, it made commitments that China will keep its word.'[17] Thus we are left with Brazil as our only hope. Brazil has consistently stood up to US and other pharmaceutical companies that have threatened to issue compulsory licences for ARVs required for its free treatment clinics. This strategy has caused the drug companies to cut their prices drastically. Thus Brazil has not yet breached any patent laws. However, as shown below, one of the largest pharmaceutical companies, Abbott Laboratories, which produces effective second-line ARVs, has now stepped into the picture. On 6 July 2006, Médecins Sans Frontières[18] issued the following grim report from Bangkok:

> People living with HIV/AIDS in developing countries who are in urgent need of an improved version of the AIDS drug Lopinavir/Ritonavir continue to be denied access to it by its sole manufacturer, Abbott Laboratories, according to the international medical humanitarian organisation Doctors Without Borders/Médecins Sans Frontières (MSF).
>
> The Chicago-based company began shipping the new formulation to a limited number of MSF projects in Africa for $500 per patient per year only after a cumbersome and time-consuming procedure. However, Abbott refuses to sell the drug to MSF for use in its programmes in Thailand and Guatemala, and has dragged its feet with registering it in developing countries. The result is that the new formulation of Lopinavir/Ritonavir remains unavailable and unaffordable for the vast majority of patients who need it.
>
> The new version of Lopinavir/Ritonavir, a second-line AIDS drug recommended by the World Health Organization, has critically important advantages over the old version, including lower pill count, storage without refrigeration, and no dietary restrictions. But without registration, the drug is virtually impossible to obtain at any price. In China, not even the old version is available, because although it is registered, Abbott has chosen not to market it in that country.
>
> 'Here in Thailand, where temperatures exceed 30°C most of the year, this drug that no longer requires refrigeration is a major advantage, but Abbott refuses to register it', said Dr David Wilson, of MSF in Thailand. 'Instead, Abbott says we can make do with the older drug that is no longer available, even on the US market, but this is clearly a second-best product and it is sold here at a price that is anyway not affordable. By limiting its $500 price to the poorest of developing countries, Abbott is adopting a policy that deliberately excludes people living with HIV/AIDS in other developing countries.'
>
> There is a growing need in developing countries for second-line regimens for patients who have been on treatment for several years. However, there is great concern that national treatment programmes and funding agencies will not be able to afford the prices of these drugs, which are much higher than those of first-line regimens. In Thailand, Abbott charges at least $2,800 for the old version of Lopinavir/Ritonavir, which means that it costs roughly ten times more to treat a patient who needs to be switched to a second-line regimen containing these drugs.

'This is a classic case of how monopolies hurt patients', said Dr Tido von Schoen-Angerer of MSF's Campaign for Access to Essential Medicines. 'We need generic competition for these newer essential drugs, because it's the only way to make them affordable and widely available. It should not be up to a CEO in Chicago to decide who has access to a life-saving medicine.'

HIV/AIDS in China

Until 2006, China was more reticent about publicly discussing its problems with the pandemic than almost any other country. This is partly due to the fact that it has suddenly found itself much sought after as a trading partner. Alarming reports by respected human rights groups have begun to filter out of the Chinese government, actually repressing domestic discussion of the issue.

Brad Adams, Asia Director of Human Rights Watch,[19] has stated:

> People infected with HIV through unsafe practice at government clinics have routinely been denied medical treatment and compensation. Now they can't even tell their story to the policy makers who might be able to help.

Human Rights Watch details widespread hostility to any kind of publicity by people with, or even commenting about, AIDS. However, the above quote referred to the imposition of house arrest of potential petitioners to the National Peoples' Congress. They were seeking redress for a government sales scheme that left hundreds of thousands of people in Hunan Province infected with HIV.

More than 20 Chinese civil society organisations reported that numerous people living with HIV/AIDS in Hunan were prevented from bringing their petition to the Congress when it opened on 5 March 2006. In fact, the repercussions were far more comprehensive than this. For instance, in Suiping County, the director of a home for children orphaned by AIDS has had to close the orphanage because of his house arrest.

The original disaster occurred when the Hunan provincial authorities encouraged hundreds of thousands of low-income farmers to sell their blood so that plasma could be made from it – a lucrative trade. When the plasma was separated from the red corpuscles, the latter were pooled and then later appropriate quantities were re-injected into the donors in order to prevent anaemia. As a result of this, HIV was just one of the conditions that were spread among thousands of people. It was reported by Human Rights Watch that the earliest of these cases of HIV were truly accidental, but that provincial authorities continued the practice even after their attention had been drawn to its effects. Eventually the national government in Beijing ordered that the practice must stop, but many provincial authorities still continued it even then. Thousands of farmers died and in some cases entire villages were wiped out. To quote from Human Rights Watch:[20]

> 'People with HIV/AIDS who are left untreated by the authorities face death sentences because they heeded the government's call for blood', said Joseph Amon, Director of Humans Rights Watch's HIV/AIDS

Program. 'The current house arrests follow earlier reports of police abuse and arrest of people with HIV/AIDS in Hunan who sought treatment and compensation.'

It was not until almost a year later that Chinese national health officials met with NGOs seeking compensation for the victims. However, when the NGOs approached the courts in Hunan for a judgement, those courts would not consider the case of anyone with HIV!

'When UN officials and outside donors are listening, the Chinese authorities consistently pledge greater openness in dealing with HIV/AIDS', said Adams. 'But their actions tell a different story. The government is silencing those most able to lead China in an effective response to HIV/AIDS, the people who are living with the disease themselves.'[21]

The Chinese official view

As is often the case, however, and without doubting the integrity of Human Rights Watch, when a country's government is confronted with a public relations problem, it often acts inadvisably at the local level while acting more rationally outside the spotlight. China's case has been not dissimilar. On 28 June 2006, the Chinese State Council established a delegation to tour around the country promoting AIDS awareness among local government officials. It is planned that at least 90% of local officials above county level will attend speeches from the delegation from 1 July 2006 until 1 January 2007, according to Wang Longde, Head of the Working Committee on AIDS Prevention and Control. He is directly responsible to the State Council.[22]

He readily admits that the AIDS epidemic in China has been rapidly worsening in recent years, and is now having a measurably negative impact in some areas. In addition, it is spreading from high-risk groups to the general public. Despite this, there are still local officials who deny the seriousness of the situation and even do their best to conceal its effects. As of June 2006, China currently has about 650,000 people living with AIDS, including 75,000 people who are actually infected.

China's growing contribution in the struggle

As we have already seen, China may yet play a pivotal role in supplying second-line ARVs cheaply through their immense potential for rapid mass production of generic copies. If that were to happen, China's comparatively late and, at times, hesitant entry into the global anti-AIDS campaign will only be a footnote in history. However, her contribution would not end there. Modern China has had a long tradition of scientific achievements since 1979, and has surprised the world yet again.

On 12 June 2006, the Chinese News Agency was authorised to release limited information on what looks like the successful development of an anti-AIDS vaccine. The details are still sketchy as I write. The following is taken from the English translation of the approved news release.

Chinese researchers say they have obtained satisfactory results through preliminary clinical testing of the safety of an AIDS vaccine developed by China.

The test concluded as the last 15 people of the 49 volunteers who were injected 15 months ago with the AIDS vaccine, China's first, on Sunday passed health check-ups at Guangxi Zhuang Autonomous Regional Centre for Diseases Control.

'Currently, data based on clinical observations have shown everything is normal, and we are confident that the AIDS vaccine is safe', said Chen Jie, deputy head of Guangxi Zhuang Autonomous Regional CDC.

'A panel of experts will make a further assessment into the experimental outcomes and decide whether to carry out the second phase of the AIDS vaccine test', Chen said.

'The assessment will cover the dose and safety of the AIDS vaccine, immunisation procedures and whether the safety of the experiment accords with the targets for clinical research set by the state', Chen said.

The Ministry of Science and Technology and the State Food and Drug Administration will decide whether to go ahead with the second phase of the test based on the assessment outcome.

The first phase of the test was launched in Nanning, capital of Guangxi, on March 12 last year, and the 49 volunteers, all Chinese and aged between 18 and 50, had received vaccine injections by October 20 last year. They were divided into eight groups. Six groups received a single AIDS vaccine and two other groups were injected with a combined AIDS vaccine. If the test enters the second phase, more volunteers will be recruited from larger groups, especially from the high-risk groups. The State Food and Drug Administration approved the first clinical phase research of the new AIDS vaccine on November 25, 2004.

China currently has approximately 650,000 HIV carriers, including approximately 75,000 AIDS patients, according to recent official estimates. We can only hope, for if it works out it will be a major blow in the fight for global equity.

The lion's share of this chapter has been devoted to HIV/AIDS, and we have not yet even touched on AIDS in the USA and the UK, as representing the developed world. However, MDG 6 referred not only to HIV/AIDS but also to malaria and 'other infectious diseases.' These will be touched upon, much more briefly than they merit, but first let us briefly survey the AIDS situation in the USA and the UK.

Life with HIV/AIDS in the USA

In 2003, more than one million people in the USA were living with HIV/AIDS, and within the next year at least 40,000 new cases were expected to be added to the list.[23] This is a rather large jump in only 25 years from 5 June 1981, when the US Centers for Disease Control (CDC), in their *Morbidity and Mortality Weekly*

Report (MMWR), published the report of five previously healthy young Californian men who developed an illness that later turned out to be AIDS.

The US health agencies responded vigorously and effectively, moving quickly through the various phases of misapprehension about the disease (e.g. that it only affects male homosexuals and it can be picked up easily, even by casual contact with an infected person's spittle) to a systematic national campaign to control it. This programme has been attended by many successes, such as the decrease in mother-to-child (prenatal) HIV transmission. The number of infants infected in this way dropped from 1,650 in the early 1990s to 144 by 2002.[24] Several preventive strategies contributed to the decline, including routine and voluntary HIV testing of pregnant women, rapid HIV-status checks of mothers, and the use of ARV therapy for HIV-infected women during pregnancy (and for infants after birth). Another success has been the widespread provision of diagnostic and screening tests for HIV.

All of these have been backed up by a heavy emphasis on sex education programmes in school and elsewhere in the community. HIV prevention strategies at all levels, from local to national – including drug treatment and peer outreach – have led to a decrease in HIV/AIDS diagnosis.[25] This has been measured among intravenous drug users in 35 areas, with HIV rates dropping from 8,048 in 2001 to 5,962 in 2004.[26] Also successful has been diffusion of evidence-based behaviour interventions (DEBIs) for HIV prevention among individuals and communities.[27] These ensure that intensive support is available to those who need it most.

Such successes not withstanding, many problems still need to be addressed because HIV/AIDS is still a leading cause of illness and death in the USA. Anywhere between 252,000 and 312,000 HIV-infected people in the USA are unaware of the fact that they are infected.[28] They are at high risk of transmitting the condition, and obviously will not be undergoing treatment.

Of course, some groups are at increased risk. For example, men having sex with men (MSM) account for 45% of new cases of HIV/AIDS, and around 54% of the cumulative figure.[29,30] About half of those in the MSM category who are infected are unaware of the fact.[31] MSM from ethnic minorities consistently have a higher prevalence of infection than their white counterparts. Between 2001 and 2004, over 35 areas, 51% of all new HIV/AIDS diagnoses were among blacks, even though the latter only represent 13% of the population. Of these, 11% acquired the condition heterosexually, whereas 54% of HIV/AIDS diagnoses in women were black women infected heterosexually. The above data were derived from the CDC's *MMWR* report dated 2 June 2006.

That excellent report also goes on to stress that DEBIs need to be increased. The present limits in this regard are attributed to staffing and financial limitations on the CDC's resources. In addition, the report mentions gaps arising from socio-cultural factors. Among these is the widespread and growing belief among sexually active young people that the problem is basically solved and they don't need to worry about unprotected sex any more! The present author, even in the quiet Sussex town where he lives, regularly encounters the same attitudes in casual discussions with teenagers. Part of this is no doubt due to the availability of treatments that did not exist until a few years ago.

It is, of course, important that schools and other outlets make effective use of those in the community who have to depend on such treatment to maintain their health. Life is no picnic for them, despite the fact that it is better than being dead. Best of all is not to be infected, and this is the message that needs to be conveyed to young people.

One could write a book about the AIDS pandemic as it affects any one country. This is especially so with a large, culturally and ethnically diverse country like the USA. However, the reader is asked to remember that the purpose of the book is to link realisation of the MDGs with health as a basic human right. The USA and especially the UK (because of its National Health Service) are in the fortunate position of being able to comprehensively address the purely biomedical aspects of the disease. However, lifestyle choices of individuals and racial and other cultural differences introduce many contextual variables. These require close study, for which this author has found no better source for the USA than the CDC's *MMWR* reports. These are accessible online and are recommended reading.

HIV/AIDS in the UK

In this account, the author intends to address issues of particular relevance to health rights and the current state of play with regard to the pandemic in the UK. To start with, we in the UK face many of the same social HIV/AIDS problems that exist in the USA. Our purely medical problems are obviously more reflective of human rights because of the broad access to diagnosis and healthcare under the NHS. However, as we shall see, even that is not as straightforward as it should be.

Throughout the 1980s, the annual number of newly diagnosed HIV infections rose steadily. It reached a relative plateau of between 2,500 and 3,000 cases from 1990 to 1998, and then began a dramatic increase again in 1999. By 2004, the annual number of newly diagnosed infections was 7,444, more than double the figure for 1999.[32] The prevalence rate is still lower than that of most developed countries, but it is rising.

There has, of course, been a precipitous drop in the proportion of new HIV cases that progress to AIDS, because of the availability of ARV drugs. This was systematised in 1996 with the establishment of *highly active antiretroviral therapy (HAART)*. This form of treatment has greatly increased the average life expectancy of people with AIDS. However, as indicated earlier, the regime for such people is far from pleasant. They have to swallow a succession of pills, some of which can cause unpleasant side-effects, for the rest of their lives. Also, as indicated when discussing second-line treatments, resistance to HAART can occur.

As in the USA, the idiotic notion that we can take a more relaxed attitude to unprotected sex, now that we have ARVs, has gained widespread acceptance among the UK's teenagers.

Treatment for AIDS under the NHS

The UK's NHS is one of the most enduring monuments to the right to health in history. Unfortunately, it does not apply to people who are here illegally. Many would argue that this in itself is a serious abrogation of human rights. However, with regard to HIV/AIDS, it is also monumentally unwise. It means, for instance, that people who have overstayed their visas, who have entered the country illegally or who are failed asylum seekers have to pay for any NHS treatment that they receive.

For the first few years after the NHS was established in 1948, this law was not in place, with the result that the UK rapidly became a Mecca for 'health tourists.' This author knew several US colleagues who spent their annual vacation in the UK having appendicectomies, etc. Therefore legislation was put in place to prevent it. Yet of course denial of treatment to, say, rejected asylum seekers can effectively be condemning them to death if the countries to which they are going to be deported are not equipped to meet their needs. In the case of HIV/AIDS, untreated people are a danger to the rest of the British community, where they may wait for months while their appeals are heard, etc. Many medical people, including this author, have signed petitions arguing that it is unethical to stop a person with HIV from receiving treatment on the basis of their immigration status alone.

This is particularly relevant in the case of HIV-positive women who are pregnant. In fact, exclusion of such people from treatment under the NHS does not only apply to various classes of 'illegal entrants.' There are certain 'notifiable diseases' for which a person will always receive NHS treatment free of charge in order to prevent contagion and epidemics. However, HIV is not on the list of notifiable diseases. If a woman has no legal right to be in the UK (e.g. because she has overstayed her visa or is an illegal immigrant), then she could (but may not necessarily) receive medication to prevent her baby from being born HIV positive. Whether or not she obtains such treatment will depend on whether doctors declare her case to be an 'emergency.'

In their annual report for 2001–02, the British HIV Association (BHIVA) included a breakdown of the gender and ethnic differences in those receiving treatment. A total of 2,044 patients from 146 centres throughout the UK were audited, of whom 73% were male, 27% were female. 68% were white, 25% were black African and 7% were classified as 'other.' In total, 44% of the patients had acquired their condition heterosexually, while 45% had acquired it either homosexually or bisexually. Around 3% of the infections were acquired through intravenous drug use. In 2004, there were 26,241 people in the UK receiving ARV treatment. More than 98% of these people were receiving at least three types of drug.[33]

Like the situation in the USA, the AIDS pandemic in the UK is generally being handled well. However, we have no cause for complacency. The growing degree of nonchalance about unprotected sex among today's adolescents is a great cause for concern, and we must be much more proactive in getting the message across. This is a community problem, and it should not simply be left to the schools. Similarly, as will be stressed in the next chapter, there can be no room for half measures. The HIV virus is indifferent to political correctness, and we cannot afford – for whatever legal reason – to have anything but universal free access to all aspects of diagnosis and treatment for AIDS for all people living in the UK.

The situation with respect to 2006

On 28 June 2006, Reuters News Agency, through its Alertnet, produced a summary of the world's capacity to contain the AIDS pandemic for the next decade.[34] It did not paint an optimistic picture, especially in the light of the 2010 target. Its report focused on a major UN meeting on AIDS, which concluded that the spread of the disease is growing, especially among women, and that the rights of the latter to protect themselves are in jeopardy. The meeting brought together leaders from 151 countries to discuss how to care for 40 million infected people between now and 2016. Since 1981, about 25 million people have died of AIDS, and 8,000 die each day. The rate of new infections has slowed down. In Africa, the rate of new infections in women exceeds that in men. At one point some Muslim countries, including Iraq, Egypt and Pakistan, had resisted any commitment on women's rights, but recently there has been some pressure to overcome this bias.

Among the 80 groups in attendance, 79 declared that the final decision was 'weak' with regard to financing health rights for girls under 18 years of age, many of them in forced marriages. Even at that, this declaration is non-binding. It points out that US$ 23 billion would be needed annually until 2010. In 2005, only US$ 8.3 billion had been spent. Despite this, the delegations did not commit to a timetable for raising the necessary funds. Oddly, it was the USA that led the objection to setting targets, even though it is the largest spender on AIDS in the LDCs.

Just as in the 2001 meeting, the 2006 meeting witnessed extreme reluctance among Islamic groups and Roman Catholic countries to make direct reference to prostitutes, homosexuals and drug addicts. The UK's International Development Secretary, Hilary Benn, told the conference that they should have been more open in their comments, and Kofi Annan's comments were similar. The US representatives explicitly declared that 'Reproductive health does not create any right and cannot be interpreted as support, endorsement or promotion of abortion.' In addition, they disassociated the Bush administration from the 1994 Cairo UN Conference on Population which had said that abortion must be regarded as a health issue and that women who have abortion must not be treated as criminals.

Despite this, though, Adrienne Germain, President of the International Women's Health Coalition, said, 'It seems that world governments are finally waking up to the fact that young people must have access to comprehensive sex education.'

In closing this chapter, it must be said that much more needs to be done about the HIV pandemic and its altogether deleterious impact on any possibility of achieving global equity in the right to health. In the next chapter, the author will consider two other conditions mentioned in the MDG, namely malaria and tuberculosis. These two major threats are momentarily hidden from many people in the developed world, for two reasons. First, HIV/AIDS grabbed the headlines, not because it had been killing Africans for decades, but because it killed five young men in California in the 1980s! Malaria has been with the human race for much longer, but has barely touched 'developed' nations. Tuberculosis is no newcomer to the developed nations. In fact, we are so 'developed' that we even thought that we had eliminated this disease among our own people! However, we really do live in one world, and bacteria are not renowned for their punctiliousness in observing political boundaries. TB is re-establishing itself as a global pandemic, as Chapter 12 will make all too clear.

References

1 Boseley S. WHO Director who led drive against AIDS, malaria and leprosy (obituary). *The Guardian*, 21 May 2006, p. 41.

2 Garrett L. The lessons of HIV/AIDS. *Foreign Affairs*, July/August 2005; www.foreignaffairs.org/20050701faessay84404/lauriegarrett (accessed 29 June 2006).

3 MacDonald TH. *Making a New People: education in revolutionary Cuba.* Vancouver: New Star Books; 1985. p. 182.

4 MacDonald TH. *Third World Health Promotion.* Lewiston, NY: The Edwin Mellen Press; 2000. p. 162.

5 Wilson L. When health education is not enough. *J Can Students Assoc.* 1990; **10**: 16–21.

6 Maposphere C, Manyeya S, Zhuwau T. *Male Condom Accessibility and Availability Within the Health Centres in Zimbabwe.* Study prepared for the National AIDS Coordination Programme. Harare, Zimbabwe: Department of Health; 1995. Available on restricted loan from University of Zimbabwe Library.

7 UNAIDS. *The Impact of HIV and AIDS in Africa. Report on the global HIV/AIDS epidemic, 2006;* www.avert.org/aidsimpact.htm (accessed 29 June 2006).

8 UNAIDS, op. cit., pp. 4–5.

9 AVERT. *AIDS in Africa: questions and answers;* www.avert.org/aids-africa-questions-1-htm, p. 6 (accessed 29 June 2006).

10 UNAIDS, op. cit., p. 2.

11 www.infochangeindia.org/healthtop.jsp?section_idr=2 (accessed 13 November 2006)

12 Reuters Foundation – Alertnet. 'India will check on UN estimate on HIV caseload'; www.alertnet.org/thenews/newsdesk/DEL73964.htm (accessed 14 July 2005).

13 Reuters, op. cit., p. 22.

14 MacDonald T. *Health, Trade and Human Rights.* Oxford: Radcliffe Publishing; 2006. pp. 15–16.

15 AVERT. *TRIPS, AIDS and Generic Drugs;* www.avert.org/generic.htm (accessed 14 July 2006).

16 Aidsmap News. 'India, China or Brazil – who will produce the second-line ARVs?'; www.aidsmap.com/en/news/24B33FA6-89-CB-42BA-88OF-1 (accessed 5 June 2006).

17 Aidsmap News, op. cit., p. 4.

18 Médecins Sans Frontières; www.msf.gr (for further information, contact: sophie.ioannou@msf.org).

19 Human Rights Watch. 'China – House Arrests Stifle HIV/AIDS Petitions'; http://hrw.org/english/docs/2006/03/11/china12879.htmp.1 (accessed 29 June 2006).

20 Human Rights Watch, op. cit., p. 3.

21 Human Rights Watch, op. cit., pp. 3–4.

22 China View. 'China to provide AIDS awareness'; http://news.xinhuanet.com/english/2006-06/28/contents_4763170.htm (accessed 29 June 2006).

23 Glynn M, Rhodes P. *Estimated HIV prevalence in the US at the end of 2003.* Paper presented at the National HIV Prevention Conference, Atlanta, Georgia, 14 June 2005.

24 Centers for Disease Control – Morbidity and Mortality Weekly Report (CDC–MMWR). *Reduction in Perinatal Transmission of Human Immunodeficiency Virus: 1985 to 2006.* Atlanta, GA: CDC–MMWR; 2006. pp. 582–7.

25 Valdiserri RO. *HIV/AIDS in Historical Profile.* Oxford: Oxford University Press; 2003. pp. 3–32.

26 Centers for Disease Control. *HIV/AIDS Surveillance Report. Volume 16.* US Department of Health and Human Services; www.cdc.gov/hiv/stats/hasrlink.htm (accessed 29 June 2006).

27 Centers for Disease Control. Evolution of HIV prevention programmes – United States. *Morbid Mortal Weekly Rep.* 2006; **55**: 597–602.

28 Ibid., p. 21.

29 Centers for Disease Control. *Fact Sheet for Men Who Have Sex With Men (MSM);* www.cdc.gov/hiv/pubs/facts/msm.htm (accessed 29 June 2006).

30 Centers for Disease Control. *HIV/AIDS Surveillance Report. Volume 15.* Washington, DC: US Department of Health and Human Services; 2003. pp. 1–46.

31 Centers for Disease Control. HIV prevalence, unrecognised infection and HIV testing among MSM in five US cities from June 2004 to April 2005. *Morbid Mortal Weekly Rep.* 2005; **54:** 597–601.

32 Health Protection Agency Communicable Disease Surveillance Centre (HIV and STI Department) and the Scottish Centre for Infection and Environmental Health. *Unpublished Quarterly Surveillance Table No. 69, 05/4.* 2006.

33 Johnson M. *Who Receives NHS Drugs for HIV?* British HIV Association (BHIVA); www.avert.org/aidsfaqs.htm (accessed 29 June 2006).

34 Reuters Foundation – Alertnet. *Nations Resist New Financial Commitments on AIDS;* www.alertnet.org/thenews/newsdesk/NO2188832.htm (accessed 30 June 2006).

Chapter 12

Malaria, tuberculosis and other infectious diseases

Malaria

As the Millennium Development Goals (MDGs) suggest, HIV/AIDS is by no means the only disease threat that we face globally. Malaria and TB are both veterans in the war against humanity, far antedating HIV. In a sense, the comparatively short period of just a few decades for which the HIV/AIDS pandemic has raged already recapitulated briefly the long history of the global spread of both tuberculosis and malaria. Let us consider malaria first.

On average, malaria infects one African child every 30 seconds. One out of every three who survive is often left with brain damage. Also particularly susceptible are pregnant women and their unborn children. Malaria is a major cause not only of prenatal mortality, but also of low birth weight and of maternal anaemia. It affects adults as well as children, and around 40% of the world's population are at risk of contracting malaria. It is no coincidence that the vast majority of these people live in the poorest countries. The morbidity figures for malaria constitute a major obstacle to social progress and equity, as it is responsible for more than 300 million acute illnesses annually, and more than a million deaths.[1]

European exploration of tropical countries, and the gradual incorporation of those countries into various European empires, have served to make malaria an important part of the developed world's history and thought. The development of malaria as a parasitic disease, both within the mosquito and then within the malaria victim, is a complex one, and it took almost a century to work out even the basic details. Such understanding, though, did gradually equip people with the means to protect themselves against infection.

To even gain a rudimentary understanding of how defence mechanisms can be elaborated against the ravages of malaria, the reader must appreciate – at least at an elementary level – how malaria is vectored by the mosquito and how the parasite responsible develops both in the mosquito and in the infected person. The strategy for fighting malaria has mainly focused on finding weak links in its complex developmental cycle – in both the mosquito and the infected person – and trying to prevent completion of the cycle.

A brief account of how malaria infection works

The parasite that causes malaria is a single-celled organism which is carried, or vectored, from one person to another by the females of various species of mosquito belonging to the *Anopheles* genus. The parasite itself belongs to the genus *Plasmodium*. Four species of *Plasmodium* can cause malaria, namely *Plasmodium falciparum*, *Plasmodium vivax*, *Plasmodium ovale* and *Plasmodium malariae*. It is

P. falciparum that causes the vast majority of malaria cases. We shall now consider the cycle, starting at the point where the mosquito bites a person and thereby injects some *P. falciparum* parasites in the 'protozoite' form.

1 Only species of mosquito belonging to the genus *Anopheles* can vector (transmit) malaria. There are 380 species of *Anopheles*, only 60 of which are able to vector the parasite. One of these mosquitoes, itself already infected, bites the person and some protozoites of the parasite pass from the mosquito's salivary gland into the person's veins. Since males of *Anopheles* species do not feed on blood, only the females can vector malaria. The males feed on plant juices.

2 In the human bloodstream, the sporozoites find their way to the liver. There they reproduce asexually – that is, by simple cell division without a need for sexual union.

3 The offspring of this asexual reproduction eventually break out from the liver cells and go back into the bloodstream.

4 In the bloodstream the following processes take place.

   a Some of the parasites (now called merozoites) then invade the red blood cells (erythrocytes), such that there is one merozoite to one erythrocyte. As the reader probably knows, the erythrocytes carry oxygen to the tissues (and remove carbon dioxide from them).

   b The other sporozoites keep re-invading other liver cells. This stage of the cycle is called erythrocytic schizogamy.

5 Inside each of the invaded erythrocytes, the merozoites undergo further asexual reproduction, eventually using up all of the oxygen in the cell. The erythrocyte then ruptures, releasing the new generation of merozoites into the bloodstream. This widespread destruction of erythrocytes results in episodes of anaemia in the affected person.

   a In some of the erythrocytes the merozoite develops into either female or male cells (gametocytes).

   b The other merozoites continue to infect more erythrocytes. This is why affected individuals typically experience chills (due to anaemia) and fever (due to the toxins released by erythrocyte breakdown) during malaria.

6 When another female *Anopheles* mosquito (or maybe the same one, if it has not already been swatted!) bites the infected person, the mosquito will take some of the gametocytes into its oesophagus.

7 The gametocytes lose their flagella and develop into spore-like structures, known as *ookinetes*. These ookinetes then invade the gut lining of the mosquito, where the male and female ookinetes combine to produce an *oocyst*.

8 These oocysts produce sporozoites by ordinary asexual cell division. The sporozoites are then carried to the mosquito's salivary gland, where the cycle starts all over again. Stages 6 and 7 constitute what is medically termed *sporogeny*.

The above cycle is summarised in Figure 12.1, which also shows how the malaria cycle includes two sub-cycles (4a, 4b, 5a and 5b).

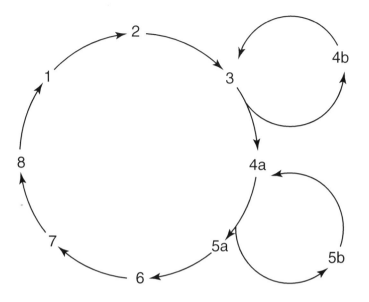

Figure 12.1 The life cycle of *Plasmodium falciparum*.

The existence of these two sub-cycles mean that, once the cycle starts in a person, infestation proceeds insidiously and quickly unless we can break the cycle at some point.

The effect on the health of the infected person can be cataclysmic and often fatal, especially in children. In Africa it would have long ago wiped out huge swathes of people if the processes of evolution had not eventually given rise to sickle-cell anaemia, which affects about 12% of West Africans.

How sickle-cell anaemia can protect against malaria

People with sickle-cell anaemia, or 'sicklers' as they often call themselves, characteristically have erythrocytes which, instead of being circular (like an automobile wheel), with raised edges and flat in the middle, are crescent-shaped instead. They are this shape because much of the complex haemoglobin structure – which is what binds molecules of oxygen or carbon dioxide to facilitate exchange of these vital gases at the tissue level – is missing. This means that the person will suffer the disadvantages of anaemia, but it will be almost impossible for them to get malaria, because the malaria parasite needs healthy erythrocytes with the full complement of haemoglobin.

The disadvantage – and it is great – faced by sicklers is that they can inherit the condition either from only one parent (heterozygously) or from both (homozygously). If they are homozygous, they are often prone to all kinds of infections, are sometimes infertile, and can die very young indeed. However, heterozygous sicklers can, if they are careful about their health, enjoy the advantage of probably avoiding malaria while remaining otherwise healthy.

In countries like the UK, which only in the last half century or so have become home to very large numbers of people of West African lineage, including Jamaicans, a percentage of sicklers is typically produced in each generation. Most people in the UK were not aware of this problem until the 1960s, when greatly increased numbers of African and Afro-Caribbean children in our primary schools made the sickler issue significant. Although the disorder has some useful functions in tropical countries with a high incidence of malaria, it doesn't have much to recommend it to the sickler living in temperate climates with frequently prolonged wet and chilly weather. However, as we shall see in Chapter 14, the geography of malaria is likely to alter dramatically due to climate change.

Historically, we have had malaria in Europe. During the first and second centuries AD, the Pontine Marshes in central Italy were breeding grounds for the right species of *Anopheles*, and malaria was common. Many of the Roman legions invading Britain had a number of malarial troops. If our climate had been such that we could get, say, a month when the temperature reached 30°C or more every day, and if the right species of *Anopheles* had been present, Britain could have experienced a malarial outbreak!

Treatment of malaria

An episode of malaria can normally be cured by various antimalarial drugs, which are much improved compared with what was available even a decade ago. The symptoms are the well-known regularly recurrent fever (every 3 days is common), bouts of extreme chills, and acute pain in the joints. However, as explained above, the cycles take place so quickly that the development of immunity to established antimalarial drugs is not infrequent. One class of antimalarial drugs consists of the chloroquines and some of their derivatives, but by 2000 whole areas of the world had developed immunity to the chloroquines. Patients in these areas now require treatment with other, more expensive drugs.

It goes without saying that if malaria had affected large areas of the developed world, disrupting production by causing high levels of absenteeism, and causing widespread infant mortality, the big pharmaceutical companies would long ago have been in keen competition with one another to find a remedy, if not a vaccine. This would have been well worth the expense and research necessary, because the victims of malaria would have been able to pay over the odds. This is very much like ARV drug research, and one wonders whether the latter would have been carried out so fast if AIDS been only an African issue.

This was well stated by the Honourable Donald M Payne in the US House of Representatives on 15 April 2006, when he stressed the importance of developing an antimalarial vaccine.[2] Although great advances have been made in this direction, a licensed antimalarial vaccine has never actually been created. A clinical trial of such vaccines is under way in Mozambique. Obviously the slow progress is due to the fact that the vast majority of people who need the vaccine are too poor to make the project profitable for pharmaceutical corporations. However, as a world community we need to make research funds available immediately, instead of waiting for kind-hearted donors like Bill Gates.[2]

And we are making progress in this direction. This author is confident that funding such as that alluded to by Payne will push one or more of the major pharmaceutical corporations to devote their energies to it. If it were to succeed, it would very much improve the prospects of ushering in the levels of global equity in human rights implicit in the UN Charter. An example of the kind of thing that fills me with optimism is a report in *Time Magazine* to the effect that the pharmaceutical giant GlaxoSmithKline has produced an antimalarial proto-vaccine for testing. The firm GlaxoSmithKline Biological in the Hospital City Clinic at the University of Barcelona in Spain, together with the Manhica Health Research Centre, announced new results demonstrating that the vaccine protects children for at least 18 months. The findings were published by *Voice of America*.[3] Even more recently, the Institute of Medicine published an announcement about the progress of two US Ministry of Health Malaria Vaccines Programmes.[4]

Funding for antimalarial vaccine research

New possibilities of funding for research and development in the area of anti-malarial vaccine production have arisen. Not only do the MDGs commit governments to increase their funding for it, but also there has been an increase in the degree to which private agencies and individuals have made substantial contributions. An impressive example of the latter has been the contribution of the Bill and Melinda Gates Foundation. If they come up with the US$ 107.6 million promised, this really will enable the Malarial Vaccine Initiative (MVI) at GlaxoSmithKline Biologicals to complete development from the Mozambique trials mentioned above. This particular programme has been given the code name RTS,S and the clear expectation is that the grant will carry the vaccine right through WHO licensing and on to African immunisation programmes. It will take time, of course – probably five years. It is important to realise that even the early stages of preparing the intended research project were funded by the Bill and Melinda Gates foundation for US$ 50 million. The project was then given another US$ 10 million in 2004, and another US$ 107 million in 2005.[5] The proposed vaccine would act on the malaria cycle at the point where the sporozoites pass from the mosquito to the person.

Another promising avenue in the search for malaria treatments is to comprehensively test drugs that earlier research had shown might be worth developing. Professor David Sullivan of the Johns Hopkins Bloomsbury School of Public Health, in the USA, has been engaged in drawing up such a list. As of 4 July 2006, the list included 2,687 drugs that have either already been approved for trial or are being tested for such approval. One of the most promising of these drugs is Astemizole, which is already widely used as an antihistamine.

Two groups of mice were infected with one of two strains of malaria – one that responds to chloroquine, and one that does not. At low doses, Astemizole reduced the number of chloroquine-susceptible parasites significantly, but was less conspicuously effective against the chloroquine-resistant strain. This represents a promising start. The Johns Hopkins Clinical Compound List is being expanded to include every drug used in clinical trials that have been approved by the US Food and Drug Administration (FDA).

Prevention – while waiting for a vaccine

Even without a vaccine, the poor of the less developed countries (LDCs) need not acquiesce to the inroads of malaria. As a white European, working in some of the worst malaria-infested areas, I have never been infected by it. Luck plays some part in this, because I had colleagues who did succumb, but judgement plays a larger role. Care in organising sleeping arrangements is critical, because *Anopheles* species are nocturnal. It is extremely uncomfortable in rural tropical conditions without electric fans or air conditioners, especially if one has to sleep and sweat under a bed-net! However, this is the best possible defence against malaria. Better to sleep fitfully in a pool of sweat, and arise in the morning untouched by malaria, than to opt for comfort and the attendant risks.

If every person. even in the poorest communities, could spend the night in a bed covered by a net, the incidence of malaria would fall dramatically. The expense is trivial. US$ 10.00 pays for one arched bed-net – that is, one with three plastic arches to prevent the netting from touching the body. There are other common-sense measures that can be adopted. For instance, the female *Anopheles* mosquito does not travel far in search of a blood meal. If the usual ideal watery breeding sites for *Anopheles* species are systematically cleared within a 50-metre radius of any dwelling, the likelihood that mosquitoes from further afield will penetrate is extremely low. They do not specifically require human blood. The blood of many other species of mammal will suffice, so the female mosquitoes are not biologically driven to hunt for human sources of blood.

In 1969, somewhat prematurely it now appears, the aim of global eradication of malaria was abandoned in favour of intensive education programmes on malaria prevention. Children who attend primary school in tropical countries are generally taught the malaria life cycle thoroughly before they go on to secondary school. The power of this small piece of education is immense, but it is only broadly effective if MDG 2 can be achieved. DDT came on the scene towards the end of the Second World War, and it really looked like a panacea that would eradicate malaria. However, within a decade the environmentally destructive effects of DDT were realised, and for this reason it is no longer in the arsenal of anti-malaria weapons.

While we await good news on the vaccine front, we need to rally all global interests to promote safe ways of living in malarial areas. The fact that the overwhelming majority of those who die of malaria are also very poor shows us clearly what must be done. If health is a 'basic human right', possession of a personal bed-net is no less of one!

An interesting possibility that will help immensely in the fight against malaria is that, given advances in meteorology, we may soon be able to predict when to expect surges in malaria outbreaks. The reader will recall that I mentioned the need for daytime temperatures not to fall below 30°C for a month for the *Plasmodium* cycle to complete itself successfully. If, in the future, meteorologists can actually predict when, where and for how long conditions ideal for malaria will prevail, we shall be in a position to predict malaria outbreaks and to prepare for them.

Tuberculosis

European civilisation lived with tuberculosis for centuries, and indeed in many instances Europeans spread the disease to areas of the less developed world that had never had it before. In Victorian times it was commonplace, especially among the poor, in large cities such as London, Paris and New York. Often referred to as 'consumption', it was long after the discovery of the bacterium responsible (*Mycobacterium tuberculosis*) that medical scientists in the developed world finally worked out how to treat it and prevent it. Starting in the 1930s and 1940s, most of the developed-world nations undertook the use of mass X-ray campaigns in schools, etc., and the use of BCG vaccination and the Mantoux test were hugely effective in dramatically reducing the incidence of TB in the developed world. The BCG vaccine is a preparation of attenuated *Mycobacterium* bacilli that, once injected into a healthy person, causes immunity to further infection. The letters BCG stand for 'bacillus of Chalmette and Guérin', referring to the two discoverers of the vaccine. The Mantoux test is a skin test which shows whether the person is already naturally immune or whether they need the BCG vaccination for protection.

Development of antibiotic-based treatment regimes after the Second World War, combined with great improvements in housing and diet for the population at large, further reduced the prevalence of TB until, by the 1970s, many health workers in the developed world began to think of it as a thing of the past. While TB was a recent memory in the USA and most of Europe, every primary school-child was made aware of how to avoid TB and its spread. Throughout the 1950s and 1960s one very rarely saw people spit in the street, for instance, because of the emphasis on hygiene in primary schools.

But how quickly we forget the lessons of history! We know that many people can carry the TB bacillus, yet not acquire the disease because they live in well-ventilated houses, eat properly, have healthy occupations and – above all – avoid infecting other people by not spitting. However, lifestyles and social behaviour have changed radically in the developed world in the last three or four decades. Spitting in public is not only ignored, but is now encouraged among teenagers as 'looking cool.' We also travel far more, and this increases our risk of exposure to infection when visiting areas where TB is still common.

In addition, only a few developed-world countries routinely check immigrants from TB-affected areas to see whether they themselves are infected. In climates like that in the UK, where for weeks at a time people may rarely go outside and/or they live in crowded accommodation, any TB that is around will quickly spread and infect. This would obviously be a particularly high risk among poorer people whose health is already at risk due to inadequate diet, etc.

The result is that, since around 1980, TB has made a sudden return visit to our big cities. It is well established once again in London, Glasgow, Manchester, Leeds and Birmingham, and easily spread by droplet infection through spitting and other antisocial behaviour. In addition, the newer strains of TB are often immune to current antibiotic treatments, so we in the developed world cannot afford to relax.

Tuberculosis in the less developed world

In August 2005, it was reported that the vast majority of TB cases (around 90%) occur in the LDCs.[6] In these countries, TB does not affect nearly as many people as malaria does, but its mortality rate is far higher. It is estimated that 1.6 million people die from TB every year. Over 35% of the world's people are infected with the TB bacterium, but only about 9 million of them go on to develop TB each year.

The disease most commonly affects the lungs, but it can attack almost anywhere (e.g. brain, bones, spinal discs). The death rate, as indicated above, is appalling. If left untreated, 50% of those who become infected will die. As one would expect, exactly as in the developed world, poverty is linked to susceptibility to TB infection. The bacterium, although it lives harmlessly in many healthy people, becomes activated in those with lowered immunity due to malnutrition, other illnesses and/or overcrowding. In the less developed world it results in a loss of as much as US$ 12 billion a year. Treatment can rarely be afforded, and in any case it takes about 6 months to work.

Because TB has also been a problem in the developed world, we are not short of increasingly effective treatments for it. Current TB drugs are so good that they are routinely effective in 95% of cases.[7] These treatments cost around US$ 10.00 per person. The leading global strategy for combating TB is a programme known as Directly Observed Treatment, Short Course (DOTS), which works to raise political awareness, and to identify and then treat TB. It is the treatment modality favoured by the World Health Organization (WHO), as it is highly effective even in cases of drug-resistant TB. Under DOTS, the drugs for the patients are free, but programme staff must observe the patient taking every single dose of the medicine for the first 2 months of the 6- to 8-month period required for the treatment. Some of the newer treatments that are being investigated also involve antiretroviral (ARV) drugs, and this readily links treatment planning to that for AIDS.

This is both fortuitous and important, for there is a close link between HIV/AIDS and tuberculosis. As the person's immune system becomes increasingly compromised by HIV, he or she is more likely to fall prey to another illness. Since the TB bacillus is so widely distributed in the population – usually inert in healthy people – it is there ready to spring into action once the body's defences are weakened. This is why TB is a common accompaniment to AIDS.

Combating TB: control of the fight against AIDS

This connection was emphasised by Dr Marcus Espinal, Executive Secretary of the WHO's 'STOP TB Partnership.' On 28 September 2004 he spoke at the University of California, Los Angeles on the cruciality of the global fight against TB. 'STOP TB' was set up in London in 1998, and one of its aims was 'to reduce the inequitable social and economic toll of TB.'[8]

Dr Espinal pointed out that the only way to stem the health crisis in Africa, India, China and the countries of the former Soviet Union is for a global fight against TB to be systematically mounted. The worst hit area is sub-Saharan Africa, where in 2004 the TB infection rate was around 300 cases per 100,000 people per year. The countries of the former USSR, China, India, Indonesia, Peru and Bolivia are close behind, with rates of 100–299 per 100,000 per year. Contrast this with Western Europe, which only had 10–24 cases per 100,000 per year. In the USA in 2004 the figure was even lower, at 10 cases per 100,000 per year.

The link with HIV is highlighted by the fact that about a third of people with HIV also have TB. Dr Espinal pointed out that women, especially those who are poor, are disproportionately denied treatment. He went on to emphasise that the WHO aimed to detect 70% of world TB cases by 2005, and to cure 85% of these. In 2004, when he made that comment, only 37% of the cases were being detected and the cure rate was 82%.

The 2005 target date mentioned by Dr Espinal was missed (as will be described later), but it did see the widening of the 'STOP TB Partnership' to include the 'Global Fund to Fight AIDS, Tuberculosis and Malaria.' Despite this, the necessity for regarding TB as the most powerful enhancer of the AIDS pandemic has not been sufficiently appreciated by many of the medical workers in the field, and certainly not by the media, in this author's view. Globally, more radical progress is being made with regard to preventing and pushing back TB in some of the LDCs than in the UK. Here I am speaking in percentage terms, of course, as the actual proportion of the developed-world population that is infected is now only about a tenth of that characteristic of the LDCs. However, unless the UK, like Denmark and the Netherlands, actually builds TB detection and remediation into its procedures for handling immigration, these statistics may suddenly change.

The global TB pandemic as of 2006

By the WHO's reckoning in 2006, TB infection is spreading at the rate of one person per second. It kills more young people and adults than any other infectious disease, and it is the world's biggest killer of women. Each year, an estimated 8 to 10 million people contract the disease, and about 2 million of them die from it. The WHO *Annual Report* for 2006 states that the Americas, South-East Asia and the Western Pacific regions will achieve their TB control targets, and that 26 countries met their targets ahead of schedule. *Global Health Reporting* issued a report on the current state of the TB pandemic, quoting the following WHO figures. The WHO estimates that in 2004 almost 15 million people were living with TB. Of around 8.9 million new TB cases globally, 3.9 million were diagnosed in laboratory tests and 741,000 of these were HIV positive. In 2004, nearly 1.7 million people died of TB, and 15% of them were HIV positive. Just over a third of people newly infected with TB in 2003 were treated under the DOTS programme. We know that active TB cases that receive no treatment can infect 10–15 people annually.[9]

A third of new TB cases currently occur in South-East Asia, but the highest incidence per capita is in sub-Saharan Africa, which also has the highest number of deaths due to TB. As has already been indicated, someone whose immune system has already been weakened by HIV is much more likely to acquire TB. TB accounts for around 13% of AIDS-related deaths worldwide, and HIV has been the most important factor in determining the increase in TB incidence over the past decade.

Between 1995 and 2004, about 22 million TB patients were treated under DOTS programmes and, worldwide, 183 countries were using DOTS by 2004. At that time, 83% of the world's population had access to DOTS in their locality. DOTS programmes reported 2.1 million new TB cases in 2004, a detection rate of 53% with an average treatment success rate of 82%. All of this amply validates DOTS as the way forward. Table 12.1, taken from the WHO Health Report 2006, summarises the matter.[10]

It was really not until the mid-1950s that we were able to cure TB with medication, but new resistant strains of the disease prevail globally. Such resistance is generally confirmed when the patient fails to complete the full course of medication prescribed and, of course, the TB bacillus cannot be rendered susceptible

Table 12.1 Estimated incidence, prevalence and mortality rates for TB in 2004

| WHO region | Incidence | | | | | Prevalence | | Mortality | |
| | All forms | | Smear positive | | | | | | |
	Number (1,000) (% of global total)	Per 100,000 Population	Number (1,000)	Per 100,000 population		Number (1,000)	Per 100,000 population	Number (1,000)	Per 100,000 population
Africa	2,573 (29)	356	1,098	152		3,741	518	587	81
The Americas	363 (4)	41	161	18		466	53	52	5.9
Eastern Mediterranean	645 (7)	122	289	55		1,090	206	142	27
Europe	445 (5)	50	199	23		575	65	69	7.8
South-East Asia	2,967 (33)	182	1,327	81		4,965	304	535	33
Western Pacific	1,925 (22)	111	865	50		3,765	216	307	18
Global	8,918	140	3,939	62		14,602	229	1,693	27

again. At first this was not taken too seriously in the developed world, where by 1960 we thought that we had pretty well eliminated the scourge. Of particular concern to health workers is multi-resistant TB (MDR-TB). This is resistant to both isoniazid and rifampicin – once powerful cures – and usually to others as well. The rates of MDR-TB are particularly high in countries of the former USSR.

The WHO is implementing its 'Stop TB Partnership' over the decade from 2006 to 2015. The intention is to achieve MDG 6 (to halt TB and begin to reverse it by 2015) in the following three stages:

1   by 2005 – to detect at least 70% of new cases and cure at least 85% of them
2   by 2015 – to reduce TB prevalence and mortality by 50% relative to the figures in 1990
3   by 2020 – to eliminate TB globally (i.e. to reduce the incidence to 1 case per million or less).

Progress made so far

Just over 50% of new smear-positive cases were detected under the DOTS programme by 2004. By 2005 it is hoped that it will reach 60%, which is short of the 70% target, but not by much.

It will be more difficult to reach the target of 85% global success in treatment, and to do this it is recognised that a sustained special effort will need to be made to increase cure rates in Africa, South-East Asia and the Western Pacific region. Seven of the high-burden countries are likely to complete the 2005 targets, namely Cambodia, China, India, Indonesia, Myanmar, the Philippines and Vietnam.

In time, if the 'Stop TB' strategy goes according to expectations, the rise in TB incidence should be reversed, and its prevalence and mortality rates halved by 2015 in all regions except Africa and Eastern Europe.

The killer diarrhoea

Although diarrhoea is particularly dreaded as a killer of babies, young children and the very elderly, it is a symptom of many diseases and can kill even young adults. John Rhode,[11] working in Bangladesh, gave the following graphic account:

> One day, seeing a patient on the porch of a headman's house in a far rural village, a man was carried to me comatose, collapsed from severe cholera. No ORT packets were available – he was on the brink of death. I asked for water, salt and sugar. They brought me a clay pot and some dark molasses and crude sea salt – all they had. Guessing at the correct proportions I hastily mixed up a solution in the pot and started spooning it into the man's slack cheeks. He sputtered and swallowed, most of the fluid flowing out of his mouth and across his chest. Patiently persisting, I managed to get a litre or so into his stomach, and he started to come around, drinking with some new vigour. In an hour he was sitting up, and we departed in my jeep for the hospital some 25 kilometres away. When I arrived there in the evening, he was walking stiffly around the ward, continuing to drink ORT to replace ongoing losses. I was a convert to 'simple solutions.'

This account gives an all too accurate picture of how rapidly diarrhoea can kill once it hits that critical point. Adults can experience diarrhoea as an annoyance and an embarrassment for two or three days before matters become critical, but in babies and young children the critical point can be reached within hours. The basic critical factor (irrespective of the pathogen that is causing the diarrhoea) is dehydration, and whether or not the rate of water loss is critical will depend on the body mass of the victim. However, treatment for diarrhoea is simple, provided that one has access to clean water, molasses (or sugar) and table salt. Because of the dehydration associated with diarrhoea, the salt, water and glucose balance is affected.

This can be remedied by administering a solution of oral rehydration salts (ORS), so long as the proportions are correctly observed. Once the solution has been prepared, it can be administered in small quantities every few minutes. This process is referred to as oral rehydration treatment (ORT). However, before discussing the details of this, we shall first consider the global impact of the condition.

Addressing illness by attacking the symptom

It is characteristic of medical workers to be suspicious – and rightly so – of medical interventions that concentrate on alleviating the symptoms of a disease. For instance, administration of powerful analgesics for the pain of cancer might reduce the pain, but will have little impact on the disease. The author once had the misfortune to visit the home of a 9-year-old girl, near Goroka in Papua New Guinea. I had heard over the radio-phone that she was suffering from severe stomach cramps, had been doing so for some days, and the parents had 'no medication.' When I got there, the girl had died of a ruptured appendix. Discussion brought out the sorry details. The girl had been unable to defecate because of the pain. The parents relieved her 'constipation' with a massive dose of castor oil and eased the pain by giving her two adult-dose capsules of Panadol hourly. Having 'no medicine' of their own did not stop them from 'borrowing' some from a local missionary! The literature is full of such dismal tales.

Diarrhoea is different, however, because most of the conditions that cause it are not themselves either lethal or long-lasting. The body often fights off the infection by emptying the bowel for a day or so to allow the healing processes to assert themselves, or else it stimulates the evacuation reflex to get rid of the transitory gut infection. If the victim is poverty-stricken, and this is the usual situation, he or she has probably not had sufficient nourishment prior to the infection, and quickly succumbs. However, if the fluid loss can be stopped, and the blood sugar and electrolyte balance restored, it gives health workers time to determine what the initial infection was and how to respond to it. The diarrhoea will not stop, but the fluid loss can be stopped.

When a child develops diarrhoea, the parents often try to compensate by giving him or her more water, but this does no good because the water rushes through the digestive tract too quickly to be absorbed by the gut. Medical workers almost instinctively favour the use of intravenous drips, which are appropriately 'high tech' and convey the confidence of professionalism. They are based on the idea of trying to avoid using the digestive tract altogether, giving the latter a chance to recover.

However, rather surprisingly, research has shown that ORT is much more effective and saves far more lives. It is cheap and does not require as high a degree of contextual asepsis as an invasive procedure, and is much cheaper. The superiority of ORT over intravenous therapy was demonstrated comprehensively in 1971, during the Bangladesh war of independence with India. The work was done under the supervision of Dr Dilip Mahalanabis of Calcutta's Johns Hopkins Centre for Medical Research.[12] During that conflict, cholera (one of the main symptoms of which is diarrhoea) swept through the refugee camps. Over 3,700 victims were treated with ORS, and over 97% of them survived. Once the fluid loss had been arrested, the patients could then be treated for the cholera itself.

Availability of ORS for ORT

Although reasonably safe ORS can be made almost anywhere, requiring only water, salt and a glucose-rich substance, it is now almost as easy to obtain small sachets of ORS which just need to be mixed with water. These contain precisely the right proportions of electrolytes and sugar and can be manufactured so cheaply (about 10 US cents per sachet, which makes a litre of the formulation) that NGOs and governments can make them widely available free of charge to affected families. Typically these sachets contain the following per litre of solution:

- 2.6 g sodium chloride
- 13.5 g anhydrous glucose
- 1.5 g potassium chloride
- 2.9 g trisodium citrate
- 20.5 g total weight of solids.

If, and *only* if, no packaged ORS is available, an emergency supply can be made using the following:[13]

- 8 level teaspoons of white sugar
- 1 level teaspoon of table salt
- 1 litre of clean water, boiled and then cooled down.

Stir the mixture until all the contents dissolve. If any readers should find themselves in the position of having to administer ORT or to show a parent how to do it, it is crucial to remember the following points, in the order stated.

1 Before handling the child, wash your hands with soap and water.
2 Prepare the ORS solution, either as described above or using one packet of ORS.
3 Wash your hands and those of the child again – because they will put them in their mouth during feeding.
4 Administer the solution in small quantities and frequently.
5 The ORS can be attenuated with other fluids such as breast milk or pure juices.
6 If the child is 4 months old or more, it must continue to have solid food as required.
7 Fresh ORS solution, whether home-made or from the packet, must be made every 24 hours.
8 Remember that ORT will *not* stop the diarrhoea, so don't worry when that persists. However, it will restore the body's compromised glucose–electrolyte balance.

9 If the child vomits, wait for 10 minutes and then start administering the ORS again.

10 As soon as possible get the child to a medical clinic.

In the case of severe dehydration, particularly of an adult, an intravenous drip may be necessary. This should only be undertaken under strict medical supervision.

What needs to be done

Unnecessary obstacles to the use of ORT still exist. This author has found that the belief is still widespread among aid workers that intravenous administration of fluids – because it costs far more and involves medical intervention – must be better. This is the case even in developed countries. A study of babies treated for severe diarrhoea at the Chicago Children's Memorial Hospital in 2003 showed that intravenous therapy costs an average of US\$ 2,299.50 per infant, whereas ORT costs only US\$ 272.78 per baby. The study did not show that intravenous therapy was better in clinical terms. Yet in the USA, 600 children who could have been saved by ORT die every year from diarrhoeal dehydration because there was no one available to administer intravenous fluids.[14]

As of 2006, the USA spends US\$ 1 billion per year on intravenous rehydration for 300,000 children who are hospitalised for diarrhoeal episodes. Around 16.5 million children suffer from diarrhoea every year in the USA. Dr Julius Goepp of Johns Hopkins University is one of a group of medical practitioners who are anxious to promote ORT, yet he quotes physicians as saying 'I like ORT, but I don't get reimbursed for using it, so I use IV treatment.'[15]

Hospitals need to change their attitude. They prefer intravenous rehydration because they don't approve of a parent holding a baby and administering ORT. Intravenous therapy doesn't require such constant accompaniment, and a busy nurse can monitor its administration to four or five children at once. Every family, but especially in the LDCs, where diarrhoea associated with various tropical diseases frequently strikes, should know about ORT. With it, even children with cholera can be saved because, with continued feeding and administration of ORT, they can be kept alive for long enough to obtain medical treatment.

This faces us with a real human rights challenge. As things stood in 2006, only 38% of diarrhoeal suffers were treated with ORT. Back in 1990, the World Summit for Children set 27 major health development goals for children to be met by the year 2000. These included a 50% reduction in deaths due to diarrhoea in children under 5 years of age, and a 25% reduction in the incidence rate. It was recognised that this would require an increase in the proportion of patients receiving ORT (and continued feeding) to 80% by the end of 1995![16] Here we are, more than a decade later, still falling short of that figure.

References

1 Millennium Campaign News. *Goal 6. Combat HIV/AIDS, malaria and other diseases;* www.millenniumcampaign.org/site/Pp asp? C=grKVL2NLEs (accessed 2 July 2006).

2 Payne DM. 'Recognition of Africa Malaria Day.' Remarks made in the US House of Representatives by the Honourable Donald M Payne (New Jersey), 15 April 2006.

3 Voice of America. *Progress Towards a Malaria Vaccine.* Broadcast 26 October 2004.

4 Institute of Medicine. *Battling Malaria: strengthening the US Military Vaccine Program.* Washington, DC: Institute of Medicine of the US National Academy of Science; 2001 (released 25 May 2006).

5 Malarial Vaccine Initiative. *Path Malaria Vaccine Initiative;* www.malariavaccine.org/files/BMFGF-Announcement-Briefing (accessed 2 July 2006).

6 Think Quest. *A Dollar a Day: malaria and other infectious diseases;* http:/library.thinkquest.org./05aug/00282/health_malaria.htm (accessed 2 July 2006).

7 Ibid., p. 23.

8 Espinal M. *Combating TB to Fight Against AIDS.* Los Angeles, CA: UCLA International Institute; www.isop.ucla.edu/article.asp?parenttid=1537 (accessed 2 July 2006).

9 Global Health Reporting; www.globalhealthreporting.org/tb.as (accessed 2 July 2006).

10 World Health Organization. *World Health Report: global TB control.* Geneva: World Health Organization; 2006. pp. 163–71.

11 Rhode J. *'Dispatches from the field: a simple solution.' Prescription for survival, global health challenge;* www.pbs.org/wbgh/rxforsurvival/series/dispatches (accessed 2 July 2006).

12 UNICEF. *Facts for Life: a communication challenge.* 3rd ed. New York: UNICEF; 2002. p. 27.

13 Rehydration Project. *Oral Rehydration Salts;* http://rehydrate.org/solutions/index.html (accessed 2 July 2006).

14 Rehydration Project. *A Solution for Survival;* http://rehydrate.org/solutions_for_survival.html (accessed 2 July 2006).

15 Ibid., p. 2.

16 Ibid., p. 17.

Chapter 13

The worldwide exclusion of minorities

The perils of belonging to any kind of minority

All over the world, there exists a particular form of systematic denial of human rights that is proving particularly difficult to even address, let alone eradicate. Ethnic and racial minorities are found in almost every country and culture in both the developed and the less developed world – for example, Romany people (Gypsies) in Eastern Europe, Kurds in Western Europe, Aborigine people in many countries, Karens in Myanmar. The list could go on. There has been a considerable move towards enlightenment in certain deeply historical forms of racism, such as antagonism towards black people and towards Jews, and this is to be welcomed. However, most nations still seem to be able to live in comfort with denial of human rights to minorities in their own country and not even be aware of it! Of course, ethnic minorities are not the only minorities – consider, for instance, sexual lifestyle minorities or religious minorities.

In this chapter we shall obviously not attempt to discuss all of the minorities that are being denied their human rights. The human mind, in its relentless search for ways of classifying people, is creative in the extreme. However, the author hopes to give a broad enough picture for us to arrive at strategies for identifying ways to recognise and remediate such violations.

One aspect that makes this issue increasingly important is that 'new' minorities are being created all the time, and at an accelerating rate, spurred on by ease of travel, and movement of refugees from the developing to the developed world. In fact, in today's world, multi-ethnic states are the norm. As recently as three or four decades ago, the idea of the 'nation state' was a widespread reality. When travelling, one encountered different traditions in food, dress, religion, politics, etc. Now globalisation has proceeded at such a pace that a bland sameness seems to have penetrated everywhere. One can stay for a few nights in a Holiday Inn almost anywhere and get by in English!

Developed-world countries have for a long time attracted people from far and wide because of their better economic prospects, and they in turn constitute little pockets of 'ethnicity' in the host country until they become sufficiently absorbed to be able to regard succeeding waves of migrants as 'foreigners.' The USA was probably the first to become famous as such a 'melting pot' in the nineteenth century, but Britain also absorbed and incorporated a long succession of ethnic foreigners, each adding their own languages and cultures to the mix. European countries such as Denmark, Norway and Sweden remained more nationally distinct for longer, but now they too are rapidly becoming multicultural societies. Out of this various ethnic and religious conflicts have arisen, but those two words – 'ethnic' and 'conflict' – need not always be seen together. For instance, religious differences, both within Christianity and between Christianity and a kind of easygoing secularism no longer excite much passion or interest. Judaism has provided another example of an easily adaptable religion over many centuries, especially when separated from its strictly ethnic definitions.

Currently there is great concern about Islam and about nationalities that embrace Islam as a state religion, but just a quick glance at history shows that much of this is overblown. When Islam started, Christianity – already 600 years old – was hardly a model of balance and compassion. In many instances it was viciously cruel and linked with the exercise of barbarous imperialism. Let us not forget that it was Islam which preserved, further developed and transmitted the hellenistic roots of the Renaissance which saved European civilisation from the dark ages.

Generally speaking, whether minorities already living in a society or new ones entering it can exist in a working relationship will depend on wise government. Denmark, Finland, the Netherlands, Norway and Sweden have, on the whole, been more conspicuously successful in this than many other countries. Of those mentioned, Finland seems to have been most successful, although of course it is not high on the list of countries to head for as an asylum seeker or refugee. In Finland, the largest ethnic minority consists of Finns whose mother tongue is Swedish (referred to as Swedish-speaking Finns, or SSFs), who constitute 5.71% of the population. The status of SSFs is exceptional compared with that of other national minorities. This is largely because the Finnish government classifies both Swedish and Finnish as official languages of the country. However, even a much smaller ethnic minority, the Sami people (representing less than 1% of the population), are well protected as far as human rights are concerned.

The Sami are the original indigenous people of Finland. They have the right to be taught in the Sami language throughout primary school, and have complete and equal access to state comprehensive schools. There is virtually no 'private' or faith-based schooling in Finland. As will be discussed later, this might be a factor that has promoted tolerance of various minority types within Finland.[1]

The government has been very much at the forefront in promoting policies of tolerance, including legislative measures that introduced higher maximum penalties for racially motivated crimes, the use of ethnic monitoring to keep track of the proportion of different ethnic groups in various types of employment, and the explicit setting of targets to increase employment to include ethnic groups that have been under-represented in various fields. A host of advisory bodies on issues such as combating racism have been created, and there has been promotion of public awareness campaigns to increase tolerance.

The author is aware of the widely held view that such strict top-down interference may actually exacerbate ethnic tensions, but his experience has suggested that the opposite is the case. Former President Dwight Eisenhower, already cited in connection with his 'military–industrial complex' speech, was concerned during the 1960s with the problems that the USA was facing with regard to racial integration in the southern states. He took the line that government interference was not the way forward, commenting that 'you cannot legislate the human heart.'[2] In fact, subsequent events proved that indeed you can, and moreover that this approach works.

Before we consider more specifics, what has the UN done with regard to creating such a context globally?

World Conference Against Racism

In Durban, South Africa, from 31 August to 7 September 2001, the General Assembly of the UN convened at the World Conference Against Racism, Racial

Discrimination and Xenophobia. This conference came about 56 years after the 1948 Universal Declaration of Human Rights. Since then racism has assumed an increasingly high profile. Many countries have enacted anti-racism laws, and human rights generally are more prominent as an issue.

Daily, technology draws us closer together, and with greater frequency. We have achieved some great victories (e.g. the elimination of apartheid in South Africa), but we have also come to know the term 'ethnic cleansing' and all the horrors that it implies. Indeed, as much of this book makes clear, our present systems of financial globalisation often lead to exploitation of ethnic minorities. Thus new tools are needed. Mary Robinson, then the UN's High Commissioner for Refugees, opened the proceedings with these words:

> This World Conference has the potential to be among the most important ever held. It can shape and embody the spirit of the new century, based on the conviction that we are all members of one human family.[3]

The agenda addressed five main themes, as follows.

- Theme 1: sources, causes, forms and contemporary manifestations of racism, racial discrimination and related intolerance.
- Theme 2: victims of racism, racial discrimination and related intolerance.
- Theme 3: measures of prevention, education and protection aimed at the eradication of racism, racial discrimination and related intolerance at the national, regional and international levels.
- Theme 4: provision for effective remedies, recourses, redress and other measures at the national, regional and international levels.
- Theme 5: strategies to achieve full and effective equality, including international cooperation and enhancement of the United Nations and other international mechanisms in combating racism, racial discrimination and xenophobia.

Since that gathering, many of the sorry events predicted and discussed at the conference have come to pass. One terrible event that had already taken place, for example, was the acrimonious and ethnically diverse break-up of the former Yugoslavia.

Fanning interethnic animosity: the break-up of Yugoslavia

The events that culminated in the savage break-up of Yugoslavia in the last decade of the twentieth century were of a horror that contradicts any European sense of 'civilised values.' They are also deeply complex, with historical roots going back centuries. This brief account will err on the side of coherence, and for this the author apologises in advance. For the sake of simplicity, I shall arbitrarily start with what befell the Kingdom of Yugoslavia – itself heaving with ethnic tensions – during the Second World War. Let it be said at the outset that although these constituent 'nationalities' occupied separate territories, this was only notionally so. For instance, Croatia also embraced significant sub-populations of Serbs, Bosnians, etc., and this was also the case with the others.

In the context of the human rights of ethnic minorities, it is important to emphasise this, because much of our modern understanding of the situation is incorrect. It is based on the assumption that, during the Second World War, for instance, some nationalities fought for Hitler and others fought for the Allies. However, this is only partly true, for each nationality included people with sympathies for the opposite side. Thus, Bosnia raised two SA divisions to serve with the Nazis, but not all Bosnians were fascists. During the war, anti-fascist partisans were led by Marshall Josip Tito. After the war, he became the leader of Communist Yugoslavia, the royalty having been deposed. He ruled until his death in 1980, and although much can be said against him, he is widely regarded as a 'political genius' in the area. It was commonly said of him that he held together a nation consisting of six nationalities, five languages, four alphabets, three religions, two ethnic groups and one leader!

Although Yugoslavia was officially 'Communist', it did not remain within the totalitarian grip of the USSR for long, and broke with it, establishing its own brand of Yugoslav Communism in the 1950s. The six republics that constituted Yugoslavia under Tito's leadership were Serbia, Croatia, Bosnia, Macedonia, Slovenia and Montenegro. In addition, there were two autonomous provinces – Kosovo and Vojvodina. Both of these were loosely under Serbian control, but their 'autonomy' within Serbia was recognised with regard to education, health and some other aspects.

In retrospect, although by no means perfect, this curious arrangement worked, and the 'minorities' tended to mix well and to intermarry. However, Tito's leadership strongly favoured the Serbs (his own nationality). Hidden behind the smooth facade of the regime, resentments were building up due to corruption, ethnic preferment, and so on. Added to this, these resentments, especially with regard to Slovenia and Croatia, were being fanned by corporate interests in the USA, the UK and Germany, who recognised advantages to be gained if these republics 'split' from Serbian control. Thus when Tito died in 1980, Yugoslavia unravelled with alarming speed. In 1991, Croatia and Slovenia broke away, seeking independence. Serbia attacked Slovenia but was quickly (and surprisingly) defeated. It then turned on Croatia, raising the spectre of religious conflict, with Serbia being largely Serbian Orthodox, whereas Croatia regarded itself as primarily Roman Catholic. All of this played into the hands of neoliberal banking interests. As indicated earlier in this chapter, the surest way to avoid ethnic conflict of this type is to exercise stalwartly fair and strong national government of such a high level of integrity that no ethnic minority feels marginalised. The Tito regime, and its Serbian base, lost sight of that requirement.

During these events, the international media played a huge role in the way that it reported news of the conflict. It is not hard to understand why Serbia, under the admittedly appalling leadership of Slobodan Milosevic, vehemently opposed neoliberalism. However, because of his own vicious cruelty in overseeing various ethnic cleansings, Milosevic very quickly lost any 'moral leadership' that he might have had in a global context. He died in 2005 whilst being tried for crimes against humanity at the International Court of Justice in The Hague in the Netherlands.

This account of the ethnic conflicts in the formerly 'peaceful' Yugoslavia is vastly incomplete. However, it does illustrate the importance of recognised standards of morality at the international level if global equity in human rights is to be achieved. In this author's view it strongly implies the necessity for a transnational body with moral authority to mediate, as will be discussed in Chapter 15. This should be the role of the UN, but as previous chapters have already shown, any moral authority that that body may have had has been severely undermined in recent decades. The interests of neoliberal finance have been allowed to prevail over human rights. This is well illustrated by the two spectacular examples of UN inefficiency, namely the conflict between Darfur and the central government of Sudan, and that in Rwanda between the Tutsis and the Hutus. Space does not permit a detailed analysis of these in this book.

The 'American Indians'

These indigenous or aboriginal peoples of North America, mistakenly called 'Indians' by early explorers or 'redskins' by many English-speaking people, have featured enormously in the European and American cultural imagination either as noble warriors and worthy foes, or as cruel and cunning to a degree. The reality is that their communities have suffered exploitation, including removal to other reservations in order to enable access to be gained to oil or valued minerals, as well as second-rate education and inadequate healthcare. The wholesale violation of their human rights continues.

Native Americans, as they are often termed, have been represented since 2000 as follows. The largest tribes, by population, are the Cherokee, Navajo, Choctaw, Sioux, Chippewa, Apache, Lumbee, Blackfoot, Iroquois and Pueblo. In 2000, it was estimated that 8 out of every 10 Native Americans were of mixed blood, but by 2100 it is calculated that this figure will be 9 out of 10.[4] However, there are also some tribes that are recognised by some US states and not others, and that are not recognised by the Federal Government. Their rights and benefits – and hence their human rights – vary from state to state. Recognition allows tribes to sell their artwork as 'Native American' and allows them access to financial support. Tribal nations that are denied any recognition include the Muwekma and Miami tribes of Indiana.[5] Even worse, many Native Americans have actually officially abrogated all of their tribal rights because such rights deny them right of probate.

Responsibility for addressing such human rights problems has been shuffled between state and federal agencies. According to the online encyclopedia service Answers.com,[6] as recently as the 1970s the Bureau of Indian Affairs was still actively promoting 'assimilation'[7] with the aim of doing away with reservations and pushing the affected people into mainstream US life. In July 2000, the Republican state government of Washington ruled that tribal governments would no longer be recognised.[8] There followed claims of theft of 'Indian' land in order to exploit the uranium and other mineral deposits beneath it.

In the US state of Virginia such disregard for human rights is enshrined in law, for in that state there are no federally recognised tribes! In 1912, Walter Ashby Plecker became Registrar of Virginia's Bureau of Vital Statistics, and promoted the passage of a law that recognised only two races – 'white' and 'coloured.' It was assumed that all Native Americans had been 'mongrelised.' Accordingly, all of the state's records of the Native American community were destroyed![9]

Notwithstanding the clearly disadvantaged status that Native Americans in the USA face with regard to such basic human rights as education and health, some attempt has been made recently in US legislation to remedy the situation.

Some of these improvements have been relatively minor, such as outlawing denigration of tribal names in advertising. Increasingly, however, Native Americans themselves have become more active in promoting their human rights in the US courts.

A more hopeful approach in North America has been evident in recent legislation passed with regard to the Inuit people in Canada.

Nunavut: Inuit territory

The Inuit people (rather improperly sometimes termed 'Eskimo') live in Canada and Greenland, but those who reside in Canada have secured a degree of autonomy not enjoyed by those in Greenland. After two decades of negotiations with the Canadian Government, a treaty was signed in June 1993 which gave them title to more than 350,000 square kilometres of land in the eastern Arctic (interested readers can access the Nunavut homepage at www.ainc.gc.ca/pr/agr/nunavut/index_e.html).

Twenty years earlier, in 1973, the Inuit Tapirisat of Canada (ITC) surveyed the boundaries of what was to become Nunavut. The land, although it covers a huge area, is all contained in the Northwest Territory of Canada. By January 1992 an agreement was in place awaiting only a plebiscite on the details of a Political Accord. In November 1992, the Inuit in the land area concerned ratified the Nunavut Land Claims Agreement (NLCA), and then on 25 May 1993 the NLCA was signed by the Canadian Government, the Government of Northwest Territories and the Tungavik Federation of Nunavut. This initiated the final stages, which ended on 1 April 1999 with the formal establishment of the Nunavut Territory and Government.

Under the NLCA, the Inuit agreed to surrender any previous aboriginal claims to any other Canadian land, and also not to assert any claim based on such. In return, they received Nunavut itself, joint membership on all management boards and CAN$ 1.17 billion to develop Inuit social programmes.

The agreement divides the land into two categories – Crown land and Inuit-owned land. On the former, the Inuits have the right to hunt, fish and participate to some extent in administration, but on Inuit-owned land the Inuits own all rights. The NLCA allows Inuits the right to negotiate with industry in non-renewable resource exploitation. The aim was to promote economic self-sufficiency consistent with the Inuits' own social and cultural needs. In addition, Inuit organisations have been granted CAN$ 1.17 billion over 15 years to develop their own social programmes.

Minority lifestyle choices and problems of human rights

These include all legal lifestyle choices that result in a minority being defined exclusively on the basis of their behaviours. For instance, although paedophiles are a minority, they do not fall into this category because what they do is illegal anywhere and contravenes the basic human rights of another group, namely children. Until fairly recently, homosexuals were also not included because the practice violated the legal codes of most countries. Research on both male and female homosexuality has conclusively established that whether or not one 'chooses' that lifestyle, the orientation itself is genetically determined. The very few studies which have not shown this are generally dismissed on scientific grounds by all leading researchers in the field.[10]

That being so, 'sexual variation' is itself a basic human right. Not only should this prevent any government from outlawing the practice itself, but (and this includes even the most 'liberal' countries) it should also prevent any country from allowing any of its organisations to restrict choice of career, say, on the basis of sexual orientation. For instance, it raises questions as to whether religious organisations can legally bar homosexuals or even women from following careers in such organisations at any level. As things stand now, however, most state constitutions exempt 'religious practices' from any such legal constraints. But is this legal under the UN Charter?

The same holds true for the practice of any kind of religion or politics that does not itself interfere with the basic human rights of its adherents – or of anyone else. Should this not apply to children under the Charter's Rights of the Child? For instance, most people in developed countries deplore the practice of female circumcision, while turning a blind eye to the circumcision of baby boys if the family's religion requires it. Why should this be so? We routinely impose many things on our children purely because it is convenient to give parents authority over them. However, looked at from a philosophical perspective, is this not contrary to the Rights of the Child? For instance, setting scalpels and direct assaults on the body aside, do I have the right to keep my children from finding out about scientific teaching with regard to the origins of life, so as to enable me to impose my religious/political perspective upon them? The author raises this not-so-hypothetical question in order to indicate the scope, difficulty and importance of the issues that we must resolve globally in addressing human rights.

Global racial discrimination

The most flagrantly obvious form of the abrogation of a minority group's human rights is based on racism. If the 'race' against which discrimination is being levelled is phenotypic (ascertainable to the eye), then the racism is easy to identify, prove and practise. If it is genotypic only (e.g. anti-Semitism), it is more difficult to identify and prove, but it is still culturally based. The UN International Convention on the Elimination of Racial Discrimination (CERD) was adopted in 1965 and subsequently ratified by 157 countries. It outlines substantive rights and a series of steps for the elimination of racism.

Article 1 of CERD defines 'racial discrimination' as follows:

> The term 'racial discrimination' shall mean any distinction, exclusion, restoration or preference based on race, colour, descent, or national or ethnic origin which has the purpose or effect of nullifying or impairing the recognition, enjoyment or exercise, on an equal footing, of human rights and fundamental freedoms in the political, economic, social, cultural, or any other field of public life.[11]

The following specific instances are taken from that same Amnesty International source.

As far as the USA is concerned, it is widely realised that even the administration of justice in that country is very much influenced by racial factors, especially to the disadvantage of black people. For instance, although blacks and whites are about equally likely to be victims of homicide, between 1977 and 2001 more than 80% of executions for murder were carried out on blacks for murders of whites. Amnesty International also records that black men are eight times more likely to be sent to prison than their white counterparts. That same ratio also holds true for black women, and Hispanic women are four times more likely to be sent to prison than their white counterparts.

Similar patterns affect the administration of justice in the EU, with a particularly strong bias against Romany people. In the EU, racial minorities of all types are generally more likely to be detained on suspicion of theft or other crimes. They also dominate the figures for deaths in custody. In the UK, police have been found to have been negligent in ensuring equal treatment of blacks and whites, and in 1999 a judicial enquiry found that the police were 'institutionally racist.'

Various social systems based on caste have built-in mechanisms for denial of full human rights to ethnic minorities. The Dalit of India (sometimes referred to as 'untouchables') are particularly well known in this regard. Indeed, in India such discrimination against the Dalit is contrary to law, but it is still widely practised. In rural areas it is not uncommon for them to experience such violations as arbitrary arrest, rape, torture and even summary execution.

Amnesty International reports that about 300 million indigenous people worldwide face discrimination and denial of human rights. State authorities regularly ignore or try to cover up such abuse. Multinational mining companies are especially guilty in this respect. For instance, in Guatemala, about 70% of the population are indigenous, and they were the major victims of that country's 'dirty war' in the 1970s and early 1980s. Despite the peace settlement that was finally achieved in 1996, discrimination still continues to deny indigenous peoples their human rights. During court trials they are not allowed to have the procedures translated.

Similarly, Australian Aborigines face real obstacles in trying to exercise their human rights. An Aborigine is 22 times more likely than a white person to be imprisoned, and is far more vulnerable to death while in custody. As already mentioned, Romany people suffer discrimination and denial of human rights in a number of countries. For instance, 'skinhead' groups seem to be able to direct racist attacks against them with impunity and sometimes even with police complicity. Women within ethnic minorities routinely suffer higher levels of such abuse than their male counterparts. There are numerous cases in point. For instance, in May 1998, in Indonesia, ethnic Chinese women were gang-raped with the support of the military. The same kind of abuse characterised recent conflicts in the Ivory Coast, Nigeria, Bosnia and the Congo, among other countries.

Kurds are regularly denied human rights in both Europe and the Middle East. We know that in the 1980s hundreds of thousands of Kurds simply 'disappeared' after police arrests. In Iraq, they have been forced to vacate the oil-rich Kirkuk region and move to Kurdish provinces in the north, so that their land can be exploited.

The ongoing civil war in Sudan continues to provide a catalogue of human rights violations against people in the south, especially the Dinka people. Thousands of them have been enslaved, and young boys have been recruited as child soldiers. As will be discussed in Chapter 15, UN agencies seem to be powerless to respond to the situation. Myanmar (formerly Burma) is another arena for crimes against ethnic minorities, especially the Karen people.

Then, of course, we have the Israeli–Palestinian conflict. Palestinian territories, under Israeli law, are treated differently from elsewhere under the same jurisdiction – with Jewish settlers being given better access to facilities, including vital medical and educational resources. Successive Israeli governments, backed and lavishly armed by the USA, are able to act with virtual impunity towards Palestinians. This became even more obvious in July 2006, when Israeli forces became engaged in fighting Hezbollah forces in Lebanon in the north, as well as the Palestinians in the Occupied Territories to the south.

Chinese authorities have denied human rights to a number of ethnic minorities – not only to the Tibetans, but also to the less well publicised Uighur people. These groups have seen their ancient cultural, social and religious rights trampled, and their political rights nullified. Any kind of public ethnic cultural expression is repressed by the government through arrests, summary executions and torture. For instance, male Uighur political prisoners have been subjected to forms of sexual torture that are unknown elsewhere.

In the EU countries, the situation is not all that much better, with reports from Austria, Belgium, Switzerland and France of brutalities inflicted on asylum seekers that would have done credit to the Gestapo. In Saudi Arabia, 889 executions were recorded by Amnesty International in the last decade of the twentieth century, and over half the victims were migrant workers.

Effects of racial discrimination in other countries

It would be beyond the scope of this book to list all of the nations in which blatant racism operates, but the following is a small sample of some of the more outstanding instances. Typically, countries or territories where such conditions prevail are themselves under acute pressures with respect to state security, etc. rendering human rights monitoring difficult.

An example is provided by Hong Kong. This 'newly recognised' area of the People's Republic of China is experiencing large-scale difficulties imposed by higher levels of immigration and by legislation that is temporarily difficult to mediate because of conflict between its former status as an international trading post under British administration, and its present incorporation into the Chinese Republic.

In 2004 it was estimated that at least 350,000 people in Hong Kong are 'ethnic minorities.' Most of them are employed as 'foreign domestic workers' (FDW). It is important for the reader to be aware of such precisely worded designations. In their case this discriminates them from local domestic workers and thus omits them from even the meagre protection that is afforded local menials. Most of these people are from the Philippines, Indonesia and Thailand. They are desperate for work and have no statutory rights. If they leave their employment, no matter how abusive their working environment, they face deportation. However, in addition to these people, about a third of Hong Kong's ethnic minorities are from Nepal, Pakistan, India, Sri Lanka and Bangladesh. Most of these individuals are employed as unskilled labourers in the building industry, restaurants, etc., and they have no employment or health and safety rights. As of 2005 there were also about 400,000 new immigrants from mainland China.

The rate of unemployment among all these groups is as high as 70% at any one time, so they face constant insecurity and are willing to do anything to avoid loss of paid employment.

The Asian Migrant Centre (AMC), a Hong Kong NGO, conducted comprehensive research on gender and racial discrimination against foreign domestic workers. It found that 60% of such workers claim that their status as domestics invites such violations, while 22% ascribed them to the fact that they were foreigners. It also found that 45% of these workers had been raped or otherwise sexually abused, 15% had been cheated out of earnings, and more than 22% were not given one rest day per week and/or other statutory holidays.[12]

As stated earlier, the Hong Kong government is itself facing extremely socially disruptive difficulties. Nevertheless, it has tried to protect the human rights of its ethnic minorities by passing a Race Discrimination Bill in 2006. However, without many international sources of support, its attempts have fallen foul of the many loopholes in the wording of the bill. These include the following.

1 Businesses are exempt for 3 years if they have fewer than six employees. However, most foreign domestic workers work for small businesses (e.g. farms, restaurants).
2 Discrimination based on inadequate fluency in Chinese is exempt from sanction.
3 Discrimination based on religion is exempt. This has mainly been used against Muslims since 9/11.

Despite this, the Hong Kong government has said that the purpose of the bill is to bring Hong Kong into line with the UN International Convention on the Elimination of Racial Discrimination (CERD). However, one crucial article in this convention requires that governments take 'special measures' to guarantee equal access to human rights. To do this, Hong Kong's government would, for instance, have to provide 'special measures' to counter such problems as higher unemployment rates and lack of access to relevant vocational training.

This is another example of the need for a transnational body to be able to force governments to create the context in which the CERD could be applied – for example, to legislate internationally for a proactive duty to promote equality. Such a positive approach may require a public-sector employer or service provider to promote equality of opportunity, for instance, or to monitor progress territory-wide in the employment of ethnic minorities.

Human rights violations in Chechnya

The fate of the Chechens well illustrates the degree to which an ethnic minority can quickly lose its human rights and become a political football in today's world. The Chechens, like the Bosnians, and before them the Sudeten Czechs and many others, have been able to suffer barbarities (and to inflict them), but in the name of a grander realpolitik that obscures moral certainties. All of this is well stated in an open letter that Eleanor Bonner and Vladimir Bukovsky, of the Society for Russian–Chechen Friendship, sent to the US President Bush in 2000.[13]

> There is nothing more dangerous in the war of ideas than the 'realpolitik' approach which has brought us so many disasters in the past. After all, was not Osama Bin Laden a by-product of a similar

marriage of convenience at one point? Was not this also true of
Saddam Hussein? And is it not true that your new 'partner', Russia,
secretly sells arms (including nuclear ones) to the 'axis of evil' countries, even now? Will the United States ever learn this lesson, or will
it forever create new enemies whilst fighting present ones?

The situation renders it easy to classify any awkward ethnic minorities who are
agitating for a level of autonomy sufficient to promote their human rights as 'terrorists.' Thus, in the recent repression by Indonesia of tiny East Timor, those
opposing them were so classified. In the ongoing struggle of the Palestinian
people – a people with no air force and hardly any army worthy of the name –
they can be defined as a 'terrorist threat' by the heavily armed and UK- and US-
backed state of Israel. In fact, the so-called 'War on Terrorism' has immediately
pushed the purely human rights aspect of ethnic minorities off the moral radar
screen in many instances.

The actual conflict between the Russians and the Chechens extends far back in
the history of both peoples. Just as the Irish Republican movement echoes centuries of colonial abuse (even mentioned by Shakespeare!), Russian literature has
featured 'Chechen' as either threat or victim for at least two centuries. Stalin even
attempted to deport the entire ethnic group to Siberian labour camps, and to physically expunge the identity of the territory. In terms of recent developments in the
conflict, US NGOs and other human rights groups (e.g. Amnesty International,
Human Rights Watch, the Moscow-based Centre called 'Memorial', the German
Society for Threatened People, etc.) have analysed the situation. In addition, some
government organisations (e.g. the US Department of State and the Parliamentary
Assembly Council of Europe) have become involved. All of these bodies are unanimous in reporting that large-scale human rights abuses are occurring in
Chechnya, and also that Russian armed forces are opportunistically committing
war crimes and crimes against humanity as defined by the UN. Breaches of human
rights law in Chechnya are far from random or accidental – they are military policy designed to undermine the Chechens psychologically. Not only is the conflict
there endangering the little republic itself, but also it is gradually impacting on the
rest of the world by its effect on the Russian authorities. In order to cover up the
abuses committed by its own military, the Russian leadership is becoming increasingly authoritarian. This in turn is exacerbating xenophobic and racist behaviour
among young people in Russia.[14]

The scale of human rights crimes committed in the conflict far exceeds any
rational response to an ethnic minority 'dispute', but without much awareness of
this by the public at large, simply because it has been reported in terms of 'international terrorism.' Vast amounts of evidence exist of other violations of the UN
Charter, such as death-squads, the creation of refugees, and lack of provision of
care and education – over many years – for the children of civilian Chechens.
Large parts of Chechnya have been turned into an ecological wasteland. Air and
artillery bombardments of oil wells, chemical plants and even radioactive sites
have caused major water, soil and air pollution. Waste products from the petrochemical refineries have been impregnated up to 17 metres into the ground. This
has caused severe pollution of the aquifers and other sources of subsoil water. All
of the above data are derived from the website of Human Rights Watch and that
of the Society for Russian–Chechen Friendship.

Attitude of the First World media

Neoliberal globalisation has not only influenced global trade in commodities, impinging as described throughout this book by its impact on human rights, but has also included almost total control of the largest media outlets. This has permitted large-scale violations of human rights to lie concealed under a barrage of news coverage about international terrorism. The Russian President, Vladimir Putin, has become adept at linking all of his actions with opposition to 'terrorism.' Thus mass terror is being inflicted on the Chechen people in the name of defending them from it! In the mean time, the West turns a blind eye in order to keep Russia 'on side.' However, the danger is that it will provoke young Muslims to give up on liberal approaches and help to drive them towards more fundamentalist solutions. Countering this, fascist and xenophobic forces among Russia's young people are increasing in a nuclear-armed country, while the West looks on.

Much has been left unsaid in this chapter, such as what happens to the minority-ethnic populations of peoples that are themselves victims of marginalisation and suppression. Hopefully, though, the material provided here is sufficient to suggest two important points.

1   Unless the human rights of any nation's minority-ethnic groups are specifically targeted for legislation at the national level, dangerous levels of alienation can occur over time and lend themselves both to domestic conflict and erosion of civic life, and to international intervention promoting neoliberal goals of global financial control.

2   Unless the UN can develop a truly transnational authority backed up by an internationally recognised World Court of Justice with actual powers, no amount of time will allow the Millennium Development Goals to be realised.

References

1 Virtual Finland. *The Sami in Finland;* http://virtual.finland.fi/netcomm/news/showarticle.asp?intNWSAID=2578 (accessed 10 July 2006).
2 www.eisenhower.archives.gov/d/LittleRock/SCHOOL.INT.pdf (accessed 20 July 2006).
3 Eisenhower D. Speech given at Little Rock, Arkansas, 4 August 1959.
4 Columbia Law Review. *Mixing Bodies and Beliefs: the predicament of tribes;* www.columbialawreview.org/articles/index.cfm?article_id=564 (accessed 10 July 2006).
5 Reference to which is found under Swarthmore College Peace Collection in the Archives of the Library of Columbia University, New York.
6 www.answers.com/topic/american-indian.p7 (accessed 10 July 2006).
7 Bureau of Indian Affairs. www.doi.gov/bureau-indian-affairs.html (accessed 12 November 2006).
8 Native American Caucus. *A Resolution by the Native American Caucus.* www.answers.com/topic/American-indian (accessed 12 November 2006).
9 *The Black and White World of Walter Ashby Plecker;* www.photoline.com (accessed 11 July 2006).
10 Moir A, Jessell D. *Brain Sex: the real difference between men and women.* London: Octopus Publishing Group; 1991. pp. 113–16.

11 Amnesty International. *Racism and the Administration of Justice; media briefing;* http://web.amnesty.org/library/index/ENGACT400282001 (accessed 11 July 2006).

12 Asian Labour Update. *Racial Discrimination in Hong Kong;* www.amrc.org.hk/5301.htm (accessed 11 July 2006).

13 Society for Russian–Chechen Friendship. *Human Rights Violations in Chechnya;* www.hrvc.net/main.htm p.1 (accessed 11 July 2006).

14 Ibid., pp. 4–5.

Chapter 14

Saving the human race: environmental sustainability

More basic than human rights

It can be argued that there is at least one thing more basic than human rights, and that is the survival of human life altogether! Amazingly, vast numbers of people and their leaders do not seem to be aware of how close we are to skating to the edge in this regard. Most readers will already be aware of the main threats to the environment – global warming, excess proliferation of greenhouse gases, pollution of vital water supplies, prodigious overuse of non-renewable sources of energy, etc. As US President George Bush so cogently expressed it, 'We are in love with oil!'[1]

Of course, debate continues as to whether or not we have already passed a 'critical point' in our country's own gradual assault on the environment, and whether anything we do now to repair the damage can make any difference. Those who take the line that we are already done for could relax, continue polluting and adopt the approach 'Eat, drink and be merry, for tomorrow we die', except that those of us who think differently might force them to restrain themselves in our own self-interest! Closely aligned with that Gothic view, some have argued that humankind really has had no long-term impact on the environment and that whatever is going to happen will be the result of long-term natural trends. Needless to say, the author does not embrace either of these views.

The issue is a big one and one which this author addressed extensively in a previous book,[2] but the situation grows more acute by the day and must be resolved as a precondition to global equity in human rights. Accordingly, for the purposes of this chapter, I propose to consider the issue under several broad categories, namely global climate change, non-renewable sources of energy, pollution, transport and trade, renewable sources of energy, deforestation, clean coal and the nuclear option. These are, of course, all interlinked.

Global climate change

Before considering the impact of climate change (loosely referred to as 'global warming') on human rights, let us consider a more basic question that is frequently raised in scientific circles, but which has so far eluded the mainstream popular media. The argument is that global climate change itself could bring about such disasters as earthquakes, floods, tsunamis, etc. Some of the more bizarre claims made after the Boxing Day 2004 earthquake and tsunami in South Asia, to the effect that global warming had gradually heated up the core of the earth to the extent that it brought about the initial earthquake, were so outrageous that many people felt that it was futile even to consider a connection. However, the basic idea is not all that absurd.

Scientists have been convinced for some time that global climate change can, and does, vary the frequency of earthquakes, volcanic eruptions, radical shifts in sea floor level, and so on. At previous points in our planet's geological history such events have come about and, according to Bill McGuire,[3] there is about to be a repeat performance. In fact, he argues that if climate change continues unheeded, we can expect not only warmer weather, but geological upheaval as well.

The earth's crust is maintained within a fairly narrow temperature range by the way in which water and ice are shifted around the surface of the globe. According to McGuire, the total pressure on the earth's crust is immense. Consider it this way. One cubic metre of water weighs a tonne, and a cubic metre of ice weighs slightly less. The coming and going of ice and water on the surface therefore results in fluctuations in pressure, thereby affecting the balance of stresses and strains on the rock formations below. These fluctuations in force are obviously most acute during periods of rapid climate change, such as we might be undergoing now. This can in turn lead to an increased incidence of volcanic activities, earthquakes, etc.

Even in comparatively recent times, geologically speaking, there is evidence of a number of such cataclysmic changes. Over the last 650,000 years alone, the polar ice caps have expanded far beyond today's limits. This has taken huge volumes of water out of circulation, holding it in enormous sheets of ice covering entire continents. Then, equally dramatically, these have melted and brought the ice back towards the poles. This activity caused large and repeated variations in sea level. All of this activity also kept varying the pressure on geological faults. As the pressure decreased, the earth's shell would bounce back in a process termed *isostatic rebound*. This would reactivate volcanic activity, leading to earthquakes and tsunamis.

Meteorologists, geologists and others are naturally anxious to find out enough of this geological history to be able to predict the advent of such natural catastrophes. Thus, in 2004, Jeanne Saunter (a geophysicist working for the US National Aeronautics and Space Administration) and geologist Bruce Molnia (of the US Geological Survey) showed that the 1979 earthquakes in south-west Alaska resulted from this 'spring-back' phenomenon. This finding has major implications for all parts of the world where glaciers and active faults coincide.

The continental shelf around Greenland is the area on which concern is focused. Imagine the impact of a tsunami starting there and sweeping south! How much destruction it would cause would depend on the amount (and speed) of global warming. For instance, the recent speeding up of the melting of the Greenland ice sheet, along with the likely collapse of the Antarctic ice sheet (especially the western part of it), mean that sea levels could rise by 5 to 7 metres over the next few centuries. This would be enough, for instance, to flood London and New York.

In the recent past, far smaller volumes of water have triggered earthquakes, including the catastrophic 1963 Mount Toc earthquake in Italy. This produced a gigantic tidal wave that easily overran the dam and wiped out the town of Longarone and took in excess of 1,000 lives. Then, in 1967, a large earthquake killed nearly 200 people in the Indian state of Maharashtra. This is now believed to have been caused by the filling of the reservoir behind the Koyna Dam. As we saw in Chapter 4, the pressure to 'develop' quickly by setting up hydroelectric projects powered by damming river systems in the less developed countries (LDCs) has already caused widespread environmental and social dislocation, accompanied by a massive assault on human rights. The considerations in the last few paragraphs suggest that we may have already initiated worse to come. It stands to reason that we cannot casually shift huge weights about on the earth's surface – which is what we do when we construct a dam – without radically changing the dynamics of the earth's crust. Indeed, it has struck this author that such vast and rapid changes could even affect the planet's orbit over time.

As we have indicated, volcanoes can also be reactivated by global climate changes. It behoves us to remind ourselves just where some of these volcanic areas are in relation to our cities. Around 57% of the world's 600 or so active volcanoes either are on coastlines or on islands just off the coast, and about 38% of them are found within 250 km of the coast. Any sudden increase in earthquake activity at or near sea coasts could bring about tsunamis that affect much of the developed world. There is also a link with the possible release of greenhouse gases, because methane gas could be freed in large quantities from the solid gas hydrate deposits trapped in the marine sediments. This could start another global warming cycle and thus accelerate the process.[4]

Of course, we cannot put every earthquake or similar disaster down to global warming, but obviously if global warming is not checked, there are likely to be more such events than there would otherwise have been. Likewise, these things tend to contribute part of a feedback cycle. Any significant increase in volcanic activity would release huge amounts of sulphate gases into the higher reaches of the atmosphere, and these would cool the earth's surface. This, in time, would temporarily slow global warming, but it is not worth waiting for. More to the point is to organise a more sustainable way of life on the only planet that we have!

Legislating for decreases in global warming

It is obvious that, as individuals, we can reduce the size of our ecological footprints in a variety of ways. At this level there has, unfortunately, been a lot of wishful thinking. As David Leal[5] rather amusingly points out, we can't fix the problem by setting up a few wind turbines and domestic solar panels, driving small cars, using high-efficiency light bulbs and taking our holidays in Torquay rather than in Greece! In fact, even now the problem is so serious that any personal solutions are going to have to be painful, especially for people in the developed countries. Attention to our individual ecological footprints is important, but the overall approach has to be much more radical and must be combined in a big way with long-term government policies at the national level, along with a high degree of international coordination of such initiatives.

The crucial point to keep in mind is that almost none of the quick fixes to the problem of carbon emissions – mainly carbon dioxide (CO_2) and methane (CH_4) – that we hear about really work. This includes such ideas as the following.

1   Planting trees to compensate for carbon emissions on a large scale. These are called 'carbon offsets.' Another common carbon-offsetting approach is the use of energy-efficient light bulbs, but at an individual/household level that does have some merit.

2 Carbon trading. This refers to legislation whereby a factory, say, is given a certain ceiling of CO_2/CH_4 emissions that it should not exceed over a given time period. If it can manage on a lower emission level, it is then allowed to 'trade the difference' with another firm that may be going over its ceiling levels. Carbon trading can also include 'offsets' from tree planting, etc.

Both of these ideas are incorporated into what is referred to as the 'carbon market.' Under the rules of the Kyoto Protocol, an international 'carbon market' exists, which includes offset projects and carbon trading. The 'carbon market' has seized the public imagination as being a 'good thing', and the big corporations like it because it confers a friendly image on what they do, while at the same time allowing them to make money out of it. However, even at the layperson level, the 'carbon market' is facing increasing criticism. One such criticism is that the 'caps' (limits) set on emissions are too high, so that not only is it easy for industries not to reach them, but also they can sell off the excess credits. In effect, this can encourage more pollution.

The basic idea behind carbon trading is that – from the point of view of global warming – where the carbon comes from is less important than the total amount. However, it ignores the fact that once carbon is in the atmosphere, rather than locked up in the ground as, say, coal – or diamonds, for that matter – it impacts on global warming. This happens as soon as we burn it. Thus carbon trading could only work – whether it is between companies or between countries – if the emissions are reduced globally (e.g. by some transnational authority) to reduce global warming. There are no easy ways to 'resolidify' it and bury it, once it is in the atmosphere as a gas. In other words, any solution that does not involve drastically reducing the use of oil and gas is unlikely to be a long-term solution. One possible answer is to use 'clean coal', as will be discussed later.

There are many other criticisms, too. For the author, the current carbon trading options exclude such polluting sectors as transport, private homes and the public sector. Flying aircraft, to transport either people or freight, is the single fastest-growing source of carbon emissions. If there was to be a really well-organised boycott of flying by the general public, along with an equally well-organised mass refusal to buy imported foods, say, the number of flights would decrease dramatically. However, this is unrealistic. Control must come from two levels before any significant improvement can be made.

1 National governments would need to set strict levels, including lowered 'caps' on carbon emissions for productive enterprises within their countries.
2 International control would have to be exercised, based on unbiased calculations of permitted global carbon emission levels consistent with reduction of global warming.

Why planting trees doesn't work

A most attractive green proposal, consistent with the 'easy-solution' approach, is the idea of tree planting. At the local and individual level there is nothing wrong with it – so long as the trees that are planted are indigenous and will be cared for. This 'greening' idea has a long history, but when large firms try to 'neutralise' their carbon emissions by planting huge tracts of trees – almost invariably pines or eucalyptus of various types – things go wrong. They cannot do it in the developed world because land prices are too high, so some LDC is targeted and a large tract of its land is commandeered, often by paying a corrupt government official, and rows of trees are then planted.

This routinely causes resentment among dislocated peasants in poor economies, with the result that – unless the forest is guarded – the trees are chopped down or burned. Even if the tree survives for its natural lifespan, it will release carbon dioxide back into the atmosphere when it dies and decomposes. In addition, non-indigenous trees can bring with them a host of agricultural and other problems. Thus tree plantations provide only temporary storage for carbon. Added to this, they take time to grow and are very susceptible (especially pines and eucalyptus) to forest fires. Pines and eucalyptus also have a far greater tendency than other varieties to increase soil acidity and to deplete the water table.

However, offset activity has now become big business and has created its own coterie of large corporations that are using the media to promote their enterprises. These firms are, of course, very sensitive to the growing political opposition to their activities, and have easily slipped into other lines of carbon offsets. One of these is the growth of biofuel material. This is certainly an improvement, but it still raises problems of space. For instance, to create any significant proportion of the fuel needed to run the UK's public transport system, acreages of biofuel plant life would be required that could not be allocated in the UK itself. Biomass is another possibility – using animal and plant waste to produce fuel.

Adam Ma-anit[6] recently produced a highly informative article on these issues in the *New Internationalist* magazine. He points out that the growing criticism alluded to above has driven the offsets industry into a complex of involvement in business beyond simple biomass and biofuel production at the local level. There is now an official offsets market, the UN's Clean Development Mechanism (CDM) under the Kyoto Protocol. More than 50% of the CDM's registered projects are in bioenergy, mostly associated with the sugar, rice, corn and palm industries. However, the issue is far from controversy-free, and has a major impact on human rights, such as land rights and genetic engineering, in several LDCs. Paradoxically, too, natural rainforests are threatened in some LDCs because of the need to clear land for biofuel production.

Corporate misleading of the public

We are aware, of course, that corporate power has from time to time been accused of misleading the public about the health implications of their activities, as was discussed in Chapter 7. However, the threat of global warming, and the reluctance of many corporate interests to acknowledge it, has led to the recent widespread use of the mass media to try to divert the public from concern about climate change.

The key message is that climate change is a good thing and only subversive elements are intent on claiming otherwise. For instance, one advertisement claims: 'They call it pollution, we call it life.'[7] This media campaign was timed to coincide with the launch of a documentary film by Al Gore, the recent US Democrat opponent to George Bush for the US President. The film, entitled *An Inconvenient Truth*, strongly promotes the urgency of global warming as a problem calling for dramatic action. Al Gore discusses the fact that the flow of ice from Greenland's glaciers has doubled since 1996, and the incidence of the most severe hurricanes has doubled in the last 30 years. He makes the truly alarming comment that deaths from global warming, if current trends continue, will reach 300,000 a year by 2030.

This is not the sort of news that the big polluter corporations want people to hear, and they have not been slow in mounting a powerful offensive against it. A group calling itself the Competitive Enterprise Institute (CEI) – largely funded by Exxon-Mobil – pays for the advertisements. They present themselves as being a freedom-loving body and hence as being anti-regulation and anti-interference with the 'market place'. This is the kind of rhetoric – regularly trotted out against the anti-smoking lobby and pro-breastfeeding groups – that paints such activists as either irresponsible idealists or politically intent on subverting 'our democratic values.'

The line that the CEI take on global warming is that it is a devious European plot to undermine US competitiveness, and they refer to the Al Gore campaign as 'the regulatory equivalent of war.' Notice how that word 'regulatory' is given an invidious connotation. As we have seen, the only way in which issues like climate change can effectively be addressed is by 'regulatory' controls – both national and global – and that, of course, would be anathema not only to individual corporations but also to neoliberal global finance itself. Reasonably educated people, both inside and outside the USA, may well find the CEI and their antics somewhat amusing, but their power is underestimated at our peril.

The CEI, and the free-market groups behind them, are in a position to influence government policy in the USA. Vice President Dick Cheney has appointed a number of Texas oil interest groups to a National Energy Policy Development Group. They are a highly secretive group, and if minutes are taken at their meeting, these are not made public. However, they have been behind the revocation of over 200 environmental laws that 'interfere' with business freedom in the USA.

In August 2005, the US administration actually announced that it would 're-define' carbon dioxide so that it no longer counted as a pollutant! Thus it could not be subject to regulation under the Clean Air Act. As another CEI initiative, the Healthy Forests Restoration Act could allow for widespread destruction of ancient US woodlands. As Alan Simpson, the Labour MP for Nottingham South, ably points out, such corporate-funded actions are designed to confuse the masses of ordinary citizens. It is not seriously intended to change the minds of scientists and environmentalists, but rather to isolate them in the popular imagination as weirdos, greenies and almost certainly 'disloyal' to great American values! This is not mere speculation. A leaked memo from the American Petroleum Institute actually included the following comment: 'Doubt is our product, since it is the best means of competing with the "body of fact" in the minds of the general public.'

There are several similar big-business 'free-enterprise' bodies in other developed-world nations, such as the UK. As any Member of Parliament knows (and, of course, Alan Simpson is one such), there is an array of similar well-financed lobby groups who make their presence felt to MPs, pushing for 'deregulation' and a 'responsibly cautious' approach to the climate change argument.

Air, water and soil pollution

Much has already been written about this topic, and there is little need to dwell on it at length here, except to indicate the respective roles of some informed lay people and statutory authorities in combating it. This is, of course, fundamental to public health and to health promotion. MacDonald[8] has described the levels of interconnectedness that must exist between the lay public and governing author-ities before people as a whole can effectively participate in health promotion. However, in the context of 'big business' and the 'freedom to choose' without regulatory interference, what chances do the community structures have?

To exemplify the situation one could find hundreds of examples, but this author has selected one from the battered city of New Orleans in Louisiana, USA. It is prominent in most people's minds because of the wide media coverage that it received when it was struck in 2005 by Hurricane Katrina, which swept over its famous 'levees' and flooded the poorer parts of the city. In that district, it was the poor and ethnic communities (in this case, mainly black Americans) that suf-fered the most, but – as such marginalised people in the USA will explain – this is nothing unusual. It didn't require a hurricane.

However, the choice of an example from the USA reflects the fact that such cases are not kept hidden by government there, because of America's noble tra-dition of a free local press. The particular case that this author has chosen clearly reflects the degree to which marginalised ethnic minorities (in this case, black Americans) bear a disproportionate share of the negative human rights impact of big business activity under neoliberalism. In this author's view, it also shows why it might well be the USA that will lead the way in implementing an alternative approach to the globalisation of human rights. Much of this optimism springs from the strong link in the USA between a free local press and the deep respect that Americans have for litigation. Cases such as the one I am about to share with the reader often involve real 'David and Goliath battles' in the courts between big business interests and the marginalised people described in the previous chapter.

Renewable sources of energy

Broadly speaking, there are five main sources of renewable energy, namely bio-mass, water motion, solar energy, wind energy and geothermal energy. We shall consider nuclear energy separately, as it cannot be classed as a renewable source. The problems that we are facing are global, rather than regional, even though it is the developed countries that confront them most immediately because of the great inequities in the use of resources by people in the developed and less devel-oped countries.

By definition, 'development' has involved confronting and exploiting the envi-ronment big time. However, much of this exploitation in order to meet devel-oped-world needs takes place in the LDCs. Since non-renewable sources of energy are finite, they will run out, at which time the developed world will have used up most of them for its own development, and global inequity will then have become 'built-in.'

Our planet, its atmosphere and all forms of life on it can potentially take up about 13.5 billion tonnes of carbon dioxide a year. If this uptake was to be equally distributed globally, then each person would account for about 2.3 tonnes per year. However, the reality is as follows. Each person living in the USA produces about 20 tonnes of carbon dioxide per year, in Germany the correspon-ding figure is about 11 tonnes, and in Japan it is around 9 tonnes. Yet these dif-ferences are trivial when compared with the situation of people in the LDCs. For instance, a person living in the Indian subcontinent produces 0.8 tonnes of carbon dioxide per year, in China the corresponding figure is about 2 tonnes and in Brazil it is around 1.5 tonnes. Can this inequity be sustainable? Suppose that all of the world's population decided to get by at the Japanese level. To do this, we would require an ecosystem ten times larger than the one that our planet currently provides!

Clearly, then, the only solution is to switch as rapidly as possible to renewable sources of energy. If we don't, the Earth may survive, but human life won't.

The potential of biomass

'Biomass' refers to any dead organic matter derived from plants as a result of the photosynthetic process. As the reader is probably aware, we all ultimately depend on energy from the sun. Animals, including humans, cannot run their bodies by accessing this source of energy, but green plants can. They do this by combining molecules of water and carbon dioxide, using solar energy directly, to make sugar in the process known as photosynthesis. Animals like ourselves eat the plants – and one another – and thereby access the solar energy second-hand. A simple equation, well known to school pupils, summarises the process as follows:

$$6H_2O + 6CO_2 - \text{(with solar energy)} \rightarrow C_6H_{12}O_6 + 6O_2$$

In other words, six molecules of water combine with six molecules of carbon dioxide, using energy from the sun, to produce one larger molecule of glucose, and six molecules of oxygen are released into the atmosphere. Thus green plants and also animals have stored a lot of carbon that was once in the atmosphere, and when they die that carbon is eventually released. Therefore biomass energy can be derived from plant or animal material – for example, wood and agricultural produce, human and animal waste. It is important to note that biomass has not been fossilised (unlike oil, coal and gas). Biomass is fresh material that can accumulate again after it has been collected.

The chemical energy that is stored in the biomass is termed bioenergy. During the conversion process (e.g. burning) the biomass releases its energy, often as heat, and the carbon is re-oxidised to form carbon dioxide. Thus using biomass as a source of energy reverses photosynthesis. If left undisturbed, biomass would slowly decompose and the carbon dioxide released would eventually find its way back into the atmosphere. However, if we use biomass as a source of energy, we imitate this natural process but at a much faster rate.

Thus the energy obtained from biomass is renewable energy. It simply recycles the carbon without adding any extra carbon to the atmosphere. Of all the forms of renewable energy, biomass is unique in that – effectively – it is simply stored solar energy.

Present-day use of biomass falls into two categories.

1 *Traditional biomass* is largely (although by no means entirely) confined to LDCs for small-scale uses. It includes fuel-wood, charcoal, rice husks, animal dung, etc.
2 *Modern biomass* is used on a large scale as a substitute for fossil fuel. It includes forest woods (e.g. rotten logs), agricultural residues, urban organic waste, etc.

Large-scale production of biomass can be used to feed into gas networks to produce heat and power. Plant oils are often extracted from plants such as rape, sunflower or oil palm, and these can then be used in biodiesel fuel. Plants such as potatoes and sugar beet, which contain large quantities of sugar and starch, can be fermented to produce bioethanol. Solid biomass can even be processed to produce hydrogen gas or methanol. However, the latter is not yet a sustainable way of producing hydrogen as a fuel, as the process itself releases large quantities of carbon dioxide.

Biomass as a source of energy has attracted some criticism. Large-scale production of biomass for industrial purposes uses up huge acreages of land that could otherwise be devoted to farming. Its processing can also result in acidification, smog and eutrophication. The latter process produces an environment that is more hostile to animal life than to plant life.

Energy from water motion

Regular water movements, such as tidal activities and river flows, can be used as predictable sources of energy. Also valuable but less predictable as an energy source is wave motion produced during storms, etc. This is referred to informally as 'blue gold.' The most well established of these energy sources is, of course, hydroelectric power.

Globally, hydroelectric power generates about 19% of electricity for domestic use and industry. In areas that are fortunate enough to have great waterfalls, comparatively little needs to be done to channel this spectacular display of energy into turbines which in turn produce electricity. However, in the absence of such natural assets, the usual procedure is to dam a river, creating a reservoir from which water is released into narrow channels (hence under great pressure) into a turbine system. As already discussed in Chapter 4, this process has many negative implications as far as human rights are concerned. In particular, as indicated at the beginning of this chapter, much of the developed world's need for energy is satisfied by exploiting the LDCs. All of the major dam projects that have been undertaken in the last few decades have been in poorer countries, often in a desperate attempt to 'develop' them so as to engage them on a more equal footing in global free trade. China is an outstanding example of this.

The clear advantage of hydroelectric power is that it is virtually pollution free, although shallow reservoirs in tropical climates can release large amounts of carbon dioxide and methane. Much can be done, though, to enhance the existing hydroelectricity-generating facilities by increasing their efficiency, rather than by building new ones. Of course, new dams will continue to be built in order to meet commitments under the Kyoto Protocol.

Solar energy

We already derive our basic life energy from the sun, but in recent years we have developed a variety of subtle ways of using solar energy more effectively. We are rapidly extending these applications at both domestic and industrial levels. Several different systems have been developed to exploit solar energy. For instance, photovoltaic modules that convert solar radiation into electricity can be built into roof tiles. Houses that were built more than 50 years ago often have roofs of the wrong shape that are sloped inappropriately for modification in this way, but there is little reason why building regulations cannot be adjusted to make it possible for most homes, and even larger institutions, to be required to use photovoltaic tiles. This would drastically cut down on fuel and electricity bills, as well as being environmentally sustainable.

Less efficient, but more generally applicable to existing buildings, is the use of solar panels to heat water in a matrix of narrow-bore pipes. In the last few years this has become popular, even in the UK. The author's cottage in rural England was built over 200 years ago, but it has been possible to install such panels on its roof which heat all of the hot water that we required for bathing, etc. It works all year round, and has rarely had to be supplemented by the existing fossil-fuel heating system. A much more expensive and elaborate system, but useful for large institutions such as hospitals and schools, is the use of solar thermal power plants. These utilise solar heat by concentrating solar radiation – using mirrors mounted on a solar power tower or parabolic troughs – and then feeding the energy generated into a turbine.

The entire global requirement for energy could theoretically be met by an area covered by 700 km² of photovoltaic cells. It is not that simple, of course, and financial considerations are the main obstacle. However, it is surprising how little use has been made of solar energy to date, with its global contribution still well below 0.1%.[9] Even given its rapid uptake, it is not expected to be contributing more than 1% globally before 2020.

An enormous additional advantage of photovoltaic modules is that they can be used to supply power in remote and sparsely populated areas where it would not be cost-effective to pipe in electricity. Not only would this be a major advantage to LDCs, which clearly cannot afford expensive power infrastructures, but also it would benefit temperate developed countries by creating the possibility of transferring power from tropical areas.

Wind energy

This author is constantly surprised by the lack of interest in the possibilities of wind energy shown by the UK government compared with, say, the governments of France, Denmark and even the USA. Great media attention is given to its negative features. For example, since wind is variable, and there are no cheap or easy ways of storing electricity, it cannot be reliable as a source of power. Wind farms are aesthetically unsightly, and proposals to build them anywhere give rise to vociferous nimbyism, industrial-sized wind turbines constitute a hazard to migratory birds, and so on.[10] However, let us consider some of the facts.

Despite the negative publicity, the wind energy business is booming and has accelerated immensely since 2000. Globally, in 1998 wind-power capacity was just above 10,000 megawatts (MW), but by 2005 it had risen to 60,000 MW. It now employs in excess of 235,000 workers.[11] In the EU, production is expected to reach 120,000 MW by 2010. Germany and Spain are now the leading European users, while France and Portugal are showing the most rapid growth rates. The advantages of wind power are obvious. It is relatively inexpensive, with costs closer to those of conventional fossil-fuel production than other alternatives. It also has huge potential for use throughout the LDCs, because its infrastructure demands are similar everywhere.

However, leading the world in terms of installations is the USA, adding 2,424 MW to their national grid. Canada has almost doubled its capacity to nearly 700 MW. Likewise, a number of Latin American countries have started to become interested, including Brazil, Cuba and Argentina. The Asian and Pacific Region countries now have a total capacity of 7,000 MW. Here India and China are the most enthusiastic users, with India already in fourth place globally. In 2005, Pakistan started to plan its first wind farm. Growth in Australia is picking up, but is still far down the league table.

The technology has also been increasing in efficiency, and wind energy production costs in 2006 are only half what they were in 1990. It has been estimated that, globally, the potential is enormous. The theoretical onshore potential alone, in sites with an average wind speed of 3 metres per second or more at a height of 10 metres, would amount to 35 times the entire electricity consumption of the world in 2006.[11]

It is this author's view that the UK needs to move more quickly in aggressively developing – and accessing – wind energy production, or even in establishing new nuclear outlets. The latter would take another 14 or 15 years.

Is geothermal energy a realistic option?

Readers will be familiar with phenomena such as geysers. These hot springs are heated from the core of the Earth, where temperatures 6,500 kilometres below the earth's crust are at around 5,500°C. The radiation of this heat is such that even the outer 3 metres depth of crust stays at a relatively constant 10–16°C throughout the year, the temperature increasing by about 3°C for every 100 metres of depth.

Geothermal energy can be exploited at two levels of intensity, namely *shallow geothermal* and *deep geothermal*. The former is drawn from the top 15 metres of the earth's crust, while the latter is drawn from greater depths. Water drawn from within the shallow geothermal level is termed *groundwater*, and it can be circulated through buildings. In winter, the groundwater is warmer than the buildings and this reduces heating costs by other means. In the same way, circulating groundwater can cool buildings in the summer, reducing air-conditioning costs. To gain access to geothermal energy, boreholes with a depth in excess of 15 metres are required.

Use of such energy involves no loss of fossil fuel. Power plants that are run on geothermal energy only emit excess steam and tiny traces of gases – at least 2,000 times less carbon dioxide than is released by fossil-fuel-run plants. They also use up far less ground space, and are 15–20% more efficient in electricity production. In addition, geothermal drilling can be undertaken almost anywhere on the earth's surface, and thus avoids the situation where one country has dominance in supply over many others.

If a geothermal heat pump is used, the savings on electricity can offset the costs of installing and running it. Where geothermal energy is used in agriculture (e.g. for heating greenhouses), such heating costs about 80% less than conventional heating. Although the use of deep geothermal energy can be costly in some places, important exceptions include the USA, the Philippines, Iceland, Indonesia, New Zealand, Mexico and Italy, where it is easily available and is therefore widely used. No doubt further research and development will quickly show how to access it at less cost elsewhere.

Cleaning up coal

We have already observed that it is practically impossible to 'repack' carbon once it has been released into the environment. Methods of capturing it and storing it underground – usually in space once required by oil or gas – have been elaborated, but at present they are prohibitively expensive. Another approach could be to develop technologies by which coal can be burned with greater efficiency (with more of the carbon being used to create heat, and less released). Encouraging progress in this regard has already been made over the past two or three decades, and includes the following.

- Washing the coal to reduce the sulphur content. This means that when it is burned, it releases far less sulphur dioxide (SO_2) and ash. The production of sulphur dioxide produces a terrible environmental deficit. When it combines with water vapour, it forms acid rain.
- Precipitation, like the famous Cottrell precipitation, electronically captures up to 99% of the ash that rises up the flumes in factories.
- Flue gas desulphurisation can reduce sulphur dioxide release by up to 97%. This process is already routinely used in developed countries, but due to the expense involved is still largely absent in such large coal-producing countries as China.

All of the above technologies, and others, have been in use for some time and are constantly being improved. For instance, it is in the interests of industries that are reliant on coal to find ways of burning it more efficiently. Some factories can now routinely achieve 45% efficiency (up from only 20% or so in the 1950s), and are looking to push it up to 50% in the next few years.

New coal-processing technologies can produce 'ultra-clean coal', reducing ash levels to below 0.25% and sulphur to only trace levels. This will enable pulverised coal to be fed directly into gas turbines, allowing it to be burned at even higher thermal efficiency levels. In addition, various gasification techniques are being developed which use steam and oxygen to convert the coal into carbon monoxide and hydrogen. This can be combined with 'sequestration', which involves dispensing liquefied carbon dioxide into deep geological strata from which it cannot escape into the atmosphere.

As things stand now, some of these technologies would incur such huge costs that private operators would not be interested in taking them on. However, the technologies will improve. In addition, many of the waste products themselves are commercially valuable. For instance, in 1999 the EU used up 50% of its coal fly-ash in building materials, with the fly-ash replacing cement, and 87% of the oxygen from flue gas desulphurisation.[12]

However, one might well ask why we should be so concerned with coal use in the light of previous observations about avoiding extracting carbon altogether as a major line of defence in preventing global warming. The answer is that, by 2010, the UK will have effectively exhausted its North Sea oil and gas reserves and will be dependent on Russian supplies of these commodities. Moreover, this very argument is being promoted by the proponents of nuclear development in support of their position. Those of us who have concerns about such problems as disposal of nuclear waste might well prefer a concentrated attempt to clean up coal, with which the UK and much of the rest of the world is well endowed.

Readers may not realise just how large a role coal still plays. About 23% of global primary needs are currently being met by coal, and 39% of electricity is generated from it. It is estimated that 70% of the world's steel production still depends on coal. Moreover, the International Energy Agency expects its use to increase by a further 40% before 2020. Without further developments in the cleaning of coal, it remains an environmental hazard. In 2000, it was producing 9 billion tonnes of carbon dioxide a year, about 70% of this from power generators. This means that 'clean coal' technology must assume great importance because, whatever else happens, we shall not suddenly switch completely to nuclear energy in 2020, even if that were desirable.[13]

The nuclear option

As far as this author can determine, informed opinions on this are about equally divided between the 'pros' and the 'antis.' The author's aversion to the nuclear option is purely strategic – if two leading experts on the relevant issue are respectively advising one to proceed and not to proceed with a certain action, ordinary survival conservatism dictates that we do not do it. It is of interest to note that the finalised rules of the Kyoto Protocol exclude the nuclear option from the Clean Development Mechanism and from Joint Implementations. However, this does not have a direct impact on any national decision on whether or not to use existing plants or to replace them. This is the situation in the UK. Of course, there are many industrialised countries that have no nuclear installations at all, and some, like Belgium, Germany and Sweden, that are phasing out their current use of nuclear power. On the other hand, Finland – a country with a fine record of responsible social policies and human rights – has adopted the nuclear option.

Finland is, of course, in many ways a very special case. For one thing, it has no significant indigenous deposits of coal, oil or gas. Yet it is a cold country with long, dark winters, so its domestic energy needs are much greater than in many other nations. However, it is also a highly industrialised country, relying upon timber processing, steel, shipbuilding, metallurgy, chemical engineering, etc. In addition, it is a large, sparsely populated country, so people have to travel long distances. Consequently, transport (both public and private) requires huge energy outlays. Finland has already used nuclear energy for about 50 years, having started planning for it in the 1950s. It started work on its fifth nuclear power station in 2002.[14]

In this chapter, therefore, I shall attempt to put forward the argument against nuclear energy, and to balance this with the arguments for it. To do this, I have read over 190 reports, papers and about a dozen books. The works of John Lovelock,[14] for instance, are highly recommended on arguments for nuclear energy. He is a renowned climate scientist in his own right and is very much aware of the need to act urgently with regard to global warming. Many readers will probably recall that he is the originator of the 'Gaia' concept, which regards the planet Earth, together with all of its surrounding layers of atmosphere and all of the life forms that it supports (including humans), as a 'living enterprise' in its own right, known as Gaia. As such, it is constantly responding – through weather, geological movements, etc. – to what is happening to it. Whether or not people survive, of course, is not its concern in balancing out its own survival forces. This is an inspiring idea, leaving our own survival very much up to what we can learn in the way of averting such disasters as unstoppable global warming, melting of the ice caps, desertification, etc. Lovelock argues that, despite its disadvantages, nuclear power is the only way forward if we are to arrest global warming.

Arguments against nuclear power

1 We have not yet arrived at a universally agreed method for the disposal of the spent rods and other nuclear waste attendant upon the running of a nuclear power station.
2 With so many small, tightly organised, violently disposed groups about – who have no objection to sacrificing themselves and anyone else around to make their point – a nuclear power station provides a splendid potential target. And no security system is perfect.
3 Contrary to much of the pro-nuclear propaganda, nuclear power is not cheap. A new installation is so expensive to build that it may well prove impossible to find enough private financers who are willing to put up the money to build one. Almost all of the countries that have nuclear power get much of the funding for it from government subsidy. Even in the USA, private funding for nuclear power stations is dwarfed by government subsidy. And, of course, the taxpayer pays for this. It is also more expensive to run a nuclear power station than to run a conventional one. When we are finished with a nuclear plant, it is prodigiously expensive to decommission it, even if this can be done with guaranteed safety.
4 Having a nuclear power station in one's country renders the country itself an increasingly likely target for nuclear attack to put it out of commission.
5 Nuclear power is not a sustainable source of energy. The amount of uranium available is finite.

Arguments for nuclear power

1 Nuclear power production produces only small quantities of waste, and these can be embedded in glass and stored deep underground. France and the USA adopt this practice.
2 Nuclear power production is not affected by weather conditions, neither does it create smog, etc.
3 The basic fuel is not expensive and the efficiency levels in deriving energy from it are much higher than we can achieve with coal, oil, etc.
4 Nuclear power does not produce polluting gases such as sulphur dioxide, nitrogen oxide, carbon dioxide, etc.
5 The security risks alluded to above can be obviated by specially trained personnel.

Thus there is no simple answer to the nuclear question. If the UK, for instance, goes down that path, it will prove a great disincentive to properly investigate or try out sustainable options. In any case, even if the Government decides to take that route, it will be at least 2020 before a new facility could be operational. Prior to that, the expenses incurred in building it will have dominated several budgets of whatever political parties are in power and undercut local community 'alternative energy' research and management. Furthermore, nuclear power is not flexible – it cannot be turned 'off' and 'on' or 'up' and 'down', and this discourages a local community response to energy needs. It places inordinate amounts of power in the hands of a few experts, and accordingly might be dismissive of public participation in decision making, etc. This cannot bode well for human rights within nuclear-powered countries.

This author must go on record as saying that he has not been convinced by all of the pro-nuclear material he has studied, much as he respects the integrity of the individuals who have produced it.

But is a solution at hand?

In closing this chapter, therefore, I refer to two more possibilities that are completely emission-free and would be sustainable for generations to come. They are: use of nuclear fusion or, alternatively, the use of Concentrated Solar Power (CSP). The former has been taught about in school science classes for years and once seemed so feasible. However, millions of pounds has gone into attempts so far to make it work. It generates energy in much the same way our sun does, by fusion of hydrogen atoms to helium, but we don't seem to be getting anywhere fast with it. Let's keep that, then, in the 'Remotely Possible' basket.[15] But CSP is a real possibility and, in fact, has been in use in California for 15 years. It is based on the idea of using huge banks of mirrors in desert areas to concentrate solar heat and convert it to electricity. Even factoring in the cost of transporting the electricity to areas where power is needed, it turns out to be much cheaper than any kind of non-sustainable fuel we have ever employed. It is estimated that as little as one half of one percent of the earth's desert area could thus generate enough energy to meet all of our global needs indefinitely and safely.[16]

We could easily embark on such a project tomorrow, given the political will. There is no time or need for despair!

References

1 Bush GW. State of the Union Address. 2 February 2006.
2 MacDonald T. *Third World Health: hostage to First World wealth.* Oxford: Radcliffe Publishing; 2005. pp. 19–31.
3 McGuire R. Earth, fire and fury. *New Scientist.* 2006; **27 May:** 32–6.
4 Ibid., p. 36.
5 Leal D. The real issues on climate change. *Morning Star,* 31 May 2006, p. 7.
6 Ma-anit A. 'If you go down to the woods today...' *New Internationalist.* 2006; **July issue:** 2–6.
7 Simpson A. Climate change is good for you – big business anti-green backers. *Morning Star,* 24 June 2006, p. 9.
8 MacDonald T. *Rethinking Health Promotion: a global approach.* London: Routledge; 1998. p. 11.
9 World Wide Fund for Nature. *Solar Energy: immense potential;* www.panda.org// about_wwf/what_we_do/climatechange (accessed 19 July 2006).
10 World Wide Fund for Nature. *Wind Energy: success story or pie-in-the-sky?* www.panda.org//about_wwf/what_we_do/climatechange (accessed 19 July 2006).

11 Ibid., pp. 1-2.

12 World Coal Institute. *Clean Coal Technologies. Briefing Paper #83;* www.uic.com.au/nip83.htm (accessed 14 July 2006).

13 Veslikansea J. *Finland's Energy Policy;* http://virtual.finland.fi/netcomm/news/showarticle.asp?intNWSAID (accessed 14 July 2006).

14 Lovelock J. *The Revenge of Gaia.* London: Allen Lane/Penguin; 2006.

15. Nuclear Fusion http://wolf.readinglitho.co.uk/subpages'nuclear.html (accessed 30 November 2006).

16 Seager A. How mirrors can light up the world. *The Guardian.* Financial Section. Monday, 27 November 2006; p. 27.

Chapter 15

Global right to health: dream or possibility?

Promises kept and promises broken

As we reach the final chapter of this book, we need to evaluate the evidence so far and draw some kind of conclusion with regard to two major issues. First, will the Millennium Development Goals be achieved? Secondly, if they will not, what alternative approaches are open to us? Any idea that the status quo is good enough hardly bears consideration. The developed world is well endowed not only with enormous financial power but also with highly articulate advocates to represent their case in global forums and to an eager media. This should not surprise anyone, for articulacy is one measure of education, and levels of education correlate positively with wealth and power. However, what might surprise some, and infuriate many more, is the degree to which one G7/G8 summit after another has promised to materially address the issue of global inequity, in particular with regard to Africa – and glibly kept deferring the issue! As I write this, the St Petersburg G8 has got under way, but so far their major preoccupation has not been justice for the deprived, but the re-emergent conflict between Israel and both the Palestinian Authority and Lebanon. Of course, it can plausibly be argued that the Israel–Palestine issue lies at the root of most of the other inequities.

Again, coming away from governments themselves, we know that the media has led billions of ordinary people worldwide to believe that they have the power to change things – the power to force the world community to unite in levelling things out. The Live 8 Bob Geldof campaign has been the most prominent case in this context. A year after the Live 8 concerts of 2005, the official report of its organisers showed that the G8 nations have delivered (and not fully at that) on only one of the three priorities it had set for itself, namely debt relief. The three priorities were debt, trade and aid. On trade they appeared to have made no adequate progress, and they have met fewer than 50% of their promises with regard to aid. For instance, it is estimated that by 2010, more than 1.5 million people who need antiretroviral (ARV) drugs and other treatments for HIV/AIDS will still be deprived of them.[1]

High finance is an arcane area for many. As we have already seen, a large number of LDCs have received 'aid' from developed countries without any money ever leaving the developed countries concerned. For instance, this can be done by requiring debt repayments to be made in US dollars, and at the same time imposing infrastructural adjustment policies by which the lender country builds the infrastructure by payment to industries in its own country. These industries make their profits, but it still counts as aid. In this context, let us consider how Nigeria had its debt cleared. The arrangement was that the Paris Club would cancel 67% of Nigeria's US\$ 30 billion debt. In turn, however, Nigeria had to pay US\$ 6.4 billion and to 'buy back' its remaining debt using oil profits. In total, Nigeria paid US$ 1 billion. This amounted to half of the aid to sub-Saharan Africa for 2005. The UK cleared US$ 3 billion – its entire African aid budget for 2004!

As Elliott pointed out in his *Guardian* article, the Gleneagles Summit represented the high point of the UK's presidency of the 2005 G8. Tony Blair, the UK Prime Minister, and his Chancellor, Gordon Brown, were adamant that African debt must be cleared, and in fact that aid must be increased by US$ 50 billion a year. Along with this, they insisted that a trade deal would be arranged to help African countries to participate in global free trade. Blair even set up a monitoring group, under the chairmanship of Kofi Annan, to ensure that the other G8 countries met their commitments. But in fact France was the only G8 country that paid up as promised. As we have seen above, the UK used debt relief granted to Nigeria (with Nigerian money!) to bolster its aid figures.

None of this is particularly reassuring. In total, if we examine the four critical areas that attracted such lavish G8 promises – debt, trade, aid and HIV/AIDS – the following emerges. With regard to debt, the G8 has delivered on cancelling 100% of debt to the 19 poorest countries. However, a further 44 countries are still waiting. On aid, the G8 promised to promote development of the LDCs by removing 'distorting subsidies' that restrict the way in which these countries organise their own economic infrastructure, for example, and to create more equitable arrangements for trade in LDC exports. To meet this target, the G8 nations promised to get rid of all import subsidies by 2013, but have so far failed to determine a method for doing so. As was mentioned in Chapters 6 and 7, present arrangements in the USA and the EU with regard to agricultural subsidies still ensure that a French cow is valued much more highly than a group of African people. In short, no reform in either US or EU agricultural subsidies is on the cards.

Looking at the situation with regard to aid is even more disheartening. The G8 had promised to double 2005 levels of aid to sub-Saharan African nations by 2010. That would have required an extra US$ 25 billion. No G8 country has actually achieved this target. Indeed, as shown above, some of them have used Nigerian debt-relief money to cover up actual decreases in aid.

Finally, with regard to HIV/AIDS, Chapter 11 presented the dismal details. The G8 promised access to treatment for 80% of the people who needed it. It is true that great progress has been made, largely due to the inspired leadership of the World Health Organization by Dr Lee Jong-Wook, but out of about 5 million people in Africa who need treatment, 1.4 million will still not receive it. When Bob Geldof and the U2 singer Bono set up the Live 8 concerts to provoke the Gleneagles G8 summit of 2005 into action, they also established a finance group to audit its impact. That audit group was called DATA (Debt, Aid, Trade, Africa), and it is from the DATA 2006 report that most of the above figures have been drawn. DATA's executive director has said that the G8 are not doing enough. They must greatly increase the pace of action if they are to achieve their 2010 targets. In particular, this means an annual increase of at least US$ 4 billion in development assistance to Africa for the next 4 years. If the G8 promises were to be kept, the impact would be enormous by 2010, with 4 million more Africans receiving the ARV drugs that they need, around 600,000 children prevented from dying of malaria, and 30 million more children going to school. Maybe just one of them would grow up to save us all from disaster.

Perspectives on the bigger problem

However, even if all of the G8 promises were kept, and indeed even if all of the Millennium Development Goals were met in full, this would not by itself guarantee that global equity in the basic human right to health would become a possibility, rather than remaining an idealist's dream. However, the material presented in all of the preceding chapters is far from reassuring even at that minimal level. A brief glance at a few global health indicators bears this out. Consider Healthy Life Expectancy (HALE), for instance (*see* Figure 15.1).

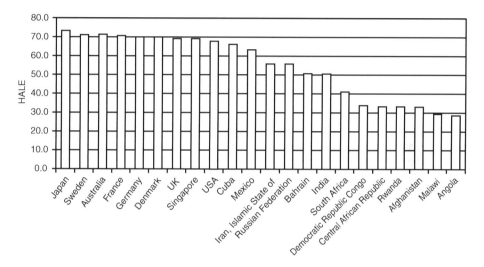

Figure 15.1   Healthy Life Expectancy (HALE) for a selection of countries, 2001. *Source:* Economic and Social Research Council (ESRC) in 2006, from the World Health Organization data for 2001.

To make sense of the chart, the phrase 'Healthy Life Expectancy' has a precise definition and it is the basic measure used by the World Health Organization[2] in its reports. HALE is only partly based on raw life expectancy, because it also incorporates a factor based on time spent in poor health. Thus it measures the equivalent number of years that a newborn child can expect to live, based on current mortality rates and prevalence distributions of health states in the population that is being examined. Stark inequalities are immediately evident from a cursory glance at Figure 15.1. For example, compare the figures for Japan and Angola. In addition, it must be remembered that within the populations of each of these countries there is variation, and this variation is greatest in the poorest and/or most war-ravaged countries.

There was a significant improvement in life expectancy worldwide during the twentieth century. In the USA, it rose from 49 years in 1901 to 77 years in 2000. In China, it increased from 40 years in 1940 to 63 years in 2000. Between 1960 and 2000, life expectancy in the LDCs as a whole increased from 46 to 63 years.[3] The eradication and/or control of infectious diseases, together with advances in agriculture, largely account for this.

However, the increases have not been universal. In many sub-Saharan African countries, HIV/AIDS has caused a decline in life expectancy, which now stands at only 47 years. Without AIDS, it would have been 62 years.[4] Similarly, since the break-up of the former USSR in 1989, male life expectancy has dropped by over 13 years to 59.9 years.[5] On a global scale, heart disease is now the biggest killer – accounting for about 13% of the total.[6,7] However, the main causes of death vary widely from one nation to another. In the African countries, infectious diseases cause higher rates of death than does heart disease. Table 15.1 compares the five main causes of death in the USA and Africa as a whole.[8]

Table 15.1 Main causes of death in the USA and Africa in 2005

Rank	USA	Deaths (%)	Africa	Deaths (%)
1	Heart disease	28.5	HIV/AIDS	20.4
2	Cancer	22.8	Malaria	10.1
3	Stroke	6.7	Respiratory diseases	9.8
4	Respiratory diseases	5.0	Diarrhoeal diseases	6.5
5	Accidents	4.3	Perinatal conditions	5.1

In Table 15.1, the inequities stare out uncompromisingly. It is clear that in Africa large numbers of people still die from diseases that have either been controlled or eradicated in the developed countries. One measure of this global inequity compares the performance of different national healthcare systems. Thus, in 2000, the World Health Organization analysed equity in access and effectiveness of the healthcare systems of 191 different countries. Table 15.2 lists the top 10 and bottom 10 countries by healthcare system performance.[9]

Table 15.2 The 10 best-performing and 10 worst-performing national healthcare systems

Top 10 countries by healthcare system performance	Bottom 10 countries by healthcare system performance
France	Sierra Leone
Italy	Myanmar
San Marino	Central African Republic
Andorra	Democratic Republic of the Congo
Malta	Nigeria
Singapore	Liberia
Spain	Malawi
Oman	Mozambique
Austria	Lesotho
Japan	Zambia

The data also reveal that 35 of the 50 worst-performing healthcare systems are in sub-Saharan Africa. Such patterns reflect national levels of economic inequality. However, the middle-income countries like Brazil (ranked 125th) and El Salvador (ranked 115th), which have higher levels of internal inequality, also perform badly. In this regard, it is surely significant that the USA only ranks 37th!

On an optimistic note, and showing a possible way forward, let us look at the progress made by Cuba with the MDGs, but especially its continued progress in pursuit of human rights in health and education. The results of the Human Development Report (*see* Table 15.3) show that Cuba is well on its way towards meeting the MDG targets in time.[10]

Table 15.3   Cuba's completion of the MDGs to date

Goal	Targets	Status
1: Eradicate extreme hunger and poverty	Halve the proportion of people living on less than US$ 1/day. Halve the proportion of people suffering from hunger	On track to be met by 2015 deadline
2: Achieve universal primary education	Ensure that children everywhere can complete a full course of primary schooling	Met
3: Promote gender equality and empower women	Eliminate gender disparity in primary and secondary education	Met
4: Reduce child mortality	Reduce by two-thirds the under-five mortality rate	Met
5: Improve maternal health	Reduce by three-quarters the maternal mortality rate ratio	On track to be met by 2015 deadline
6: Combat HIV/AIDS, malaria and other diseases	Have halted by 2015 and begun to reverse the spread of HIV/AIDS. Have halted by 2015 and begun to reverse the incidence of malaria and other major diseases	On track to be met by 2015 deadline
7: Ensure environmental sustainability	Integrate sustainable development principles into country policies, and reverse loss of environmental resources. Halve the proportion of people without sustainable access to safe drinking water and sanitation. By 2020, achieve a significant improvement in the lives of at least 100 million slum dwellers. Develop further an open, rule-based, predictable, non-discriminatory trading and financial system. Address the special needs of the LDCs. Address the special needs of landlocked countries and small island developing states.	Potential to be met by 2015 deadline
8: Develop a global partnership for development	Deal comprehensively with the debt problems of developing countries through national and international measures in order to make debt sustainable in the long term.	Potential to be met by 2015 deadline

Table 15.3   (Continued)

Goal	Targets	Status
	Develop and implement strategies for decent and productive work for young people. Provide access to affordable essential drugs in developing countries. Make available the benefits of new technologies, especially information and communication.	

Source: Human Development Report 2005.[10]

Alternatives to neoliberal financial globalisation

As has already been stated in this book, neoliberalism is not an American invention, nor is the US hegemony in the system guaranteed. Much opposition to it comes from thoughtful US citizens and, in addition, the rules of neoliberal finance can be just as efficiently used by other nationalities. Nor is the basic problem globalised trade and globalised finance itself. The only possible solution, if equity in health is to be achieved, is a globalised finance system. The real issue is how this can be mediated without forcing the UN into its present self-contradictory position of ruling on international human rights while at the same time running agencies that sustain the violation of those rights. This is well argued by the Nobel Prize-winning economist, Joseph Stiglitz.[11]

Increasingly, people are becoming aware that the much-vaunted 'freedom' of current competitive, market-dominated, neoliberalism harbours reserves of violence that periodically erupt as wars. Like any competition, it produces winners (and that is its attraction), but it must also produce losers, and they are as integral a part of the system as the winners. We cannot merely say that the losers are a blip on the system and that fine-tuning the whole apparatus will gradually fade them out of the picture. Without the losers the system wouldn't work.

Evidence from the real world is utterly compelling in this regard. Prosperity, even for the majority of the world's people, let alone all of them, under neoliberalism has to be an empty promise. The former chairman of the US Federal Reserve Board, the economist Alan Greenspan, frequently used the term 'hegemony' to describe US financial and structural global dominance. One imagines that this did not go down too well with other nations. China, for instance, might be anxious to assume that level of leadership. However, Greenspan's remarks showed that he realised that politics does not deal only (or maybe at all) with moral validity, but with naked power. The ideology of neoliberalism is persuasive because it is backed up by enormous military power. In a sense, it is able to construct its own version of 'reality' and this appears, as has been observed by Shan Saeed,[12] to be both internally consistent and theoretically rational. In effect, it puts forward a false economy along the following lines. Poverty and degradation are indeed unfortunate, but they are preferable to outright starvation. These are presented as the only alternatives for human rights. The World Bank itself has estimated that neoliberal globalisation created 200 million new poor people between 1993 and 2003.[13] However, this does not prevent most of the media from proclaiming that neoliberalism is the only hope for global prosperity, and millions of lay people from accepting that as an article of faith. Therefore, let us look at the Chinese situation.

Bases for Chinese global financial hegemony

As was suggested in Chapter 1, neoliberalism does not require US hegemony. The same system, or one very similar to it, can be assumed by another nation. The big problem, from the point of view of continued US financial hegemony, is the basic rules enunciated at the Bretton Woods Conference in 1944, when it was insisted that all international transactions had to take place in US dollars. In doing that, it has created a global finance based on the ease with which US dollars can mediate financial activity all over the world, but *without* a corresponding free movement of labour forces. Over time, this has created huge increases in the numbers of asylum seekers and illegal immigrants, and in the trafficking of prostitutes. As the author has observed previously,[14] if a wealthy nation's enterprises enter into a poorer country and carry off its resources, the people will try to follow the loot. In that sense, it can even be argued that the current system of neoliberal financial domination by the USA is not truly globalisation because it is only moving US dollars but not the labour forces that generate them.

In his article, Shan Saeed points out that the dollar hegemony involves the USA producing the dollars while the rest of the world creates the goods and services that are traded for the dollars. As was mentioned in Chapter 3, as the oil crisis started to get under way in 1971, US president Richard Nixon abandoned the gold reserve system, instead adjusting exchange rates to stop gold draining from the US Treasury. This was being caused by frequent lapses of US fiscal control over trade in dollars. Some saw this as the US dollar giving up as a reserve currency for international trade, but in fact quite the opposite was happening. The dollar has remained as the only reserve currency for world trade, despite the fact that accelerating US trade deficits have made the USA the world's most indebted nation.

Nixon's strategy may have seemed wise at the time, but what is to stop China, say, from making the yuan an alternative world currency by demanding that all trade with China be mediated in this way? It clearly has a large enough global trade network for such an action to succeed. If the Chinese government made it illegal for Chinese exporters to accept payment in other currencies, and announced that all Chinese exports must be paid for in yuan, there would be a concerted drive by all countries buying Chinese goods to purchase yuan. And business firms that already had yuan as their currency would no longer have to exchange it for dollars – currently a source of profit for the USA. The die would be well and truly cast once the OPEC countries accepted yuan, instead of dollars, for oil. This could easily be sustained by China's enormous export growth since the late 1990s. As the reader will recall, that came about at the expense of the now wounded South-East Asian economies. These former 'Tiger Economies' are now trapped in long-term financial difficulties because of huge foreign-currency debts, and have had to call increasingly on the IMF for bailout loans. This is of course agreeable to US banks, who profit from the harsher than usual SAPs to protect their G8 creditors. It allows the USA, for now, to break down traditionally impregnable financial systems in one Asian country after another, starting with South Korea, Japan and India.

This 'stealth by structural adjustment' is surely intended to dismantle domestically controlled Asian economies and to replace them with a global system controlled by the USA. Of course, the real US target is China. However, the Chinese economy has very quickly become internationally valued in such important fields as telecommunications, medical technology, aerospace and electronics, with all of their potential for military application. Moreover, this implicit potential of the 'sleeping giant' of China has enormous human resources behind it. In universities in the EU and the USA there has been a dramatic increase in the proportion of Chinese students. Little can now prevent China from becoming the leading producer of brain power to steer its own globally spread technology.[15]

All of this will make China a preferred alternative trading power for other Asian countries. If this can be achieved with more mutually advantageous trading arrangements on a basis of 'regional fair trade',[16] rather than WTO-dominated 'free trade', globalised finance will inevitably undergo a change of hegemony, and Alan Greenspan may, in his retirement years, regret his unfortunately over-confident turn of phrase. Of course, any such drastic shift – no matter how 'economically inevitable' – would be resisted by US interests.

One possibly Gothic scenario that worries this author is that the present US administration, aware of its precarious economic position, may be undertaking some kind of endgame in the Middle East, using Israel as its pawn. If, say, Iraq and Iran (plus minor inputs from the Palestinian Authority and Lebanon) can be brought into conflict with Israel, that would give the US military an opportunity to try out the feasibility of tactical nuclear weapons.[a] At the same time they could gain control over the huge Middle Eastern oil resources which they so badly need.

The growing context for alternatives to neoliberalism

The very difficulties that are now being experienced worldwide – and even within the USA and EU – with neoliberalism as a social policy, provide an ever increasing context for new ideas. Present power politics would like people to believe that neoliberalism is the only reality and that we have to learn to live with it and to find ways of adjusting our moral concerns to it. That view has been widely articulated, but perhaps the best expressed such account is by Jonathan Porritt.[17]

Much of the recent objection to neoliberalism has emerged as a 'gut-level' response to the impact on many LDCs, especially in Africa, of the economic policies of the World Bank and the IMF, and of the pro-corporate interventions by the WTO. Such inhumane policies have undermined the economies of nations such as Mexico, Brazil and Ecuador, and this has provoked social scientists to analyse the long-term consequences of the free-market system. However, it would be a mistake to assume that the developed nations – even the powerful G8 nations – have escaped its impacts or that this has not attracted scholarly analysis. Even as far back as the 1960s, during the 'optimistic' Kennedy era in the USA, it was certainly clear internationally that neoliberal trade policies were alienating much opinion in Latin America, Asia and Africa. In the USA itself, things became conspicuously worse during the Richard Nixon presidency, and then with the

inauguration of Ronald Reagan. It was then that, on the one hand, the destruction of the US welfare state and other assaults on American civic life, and on the
other, a noticeable shift to the right of the media, really became evident to
thoughtful Americans. They witnessed a marked increase in the creation of
domestic prison–industrial complexes,[18] and the increasingly flagrant use of the
US military in a variety of LDCs.

The literature suggests that Americans who discuss the power of neoliberalism
in daily US life are likely to perpetuate the idea that 'free markets' and con-
sumerism are the only real guarantors of 'freedom.' They are liable to be vocal
about classifying ideas of improving the situation or, God forbid, of egalitarian
utopias, as utterly absurd and 'unrealistic.' However, the true 'unrealism' is the
belief that political democracy can exist without economic democracy. Let us look
at the 'real' situation both in the USA and globally.

In Iraq, the USA has got itself deeper and deeper into a no-win situation. At
the time of writing, over 2,000 US soldiers have been killed, with estimates that
there have been over 100,000 Iraqi civilian deaths. Israel continues to construct
a concrete wall over nine feet tall over swathes of Palestinian territory. Back in
1995, when the WTO was founded, it seemed to many people that neoliberalism
was the only honest answer, and that people who adopted a contrary view were
either confused Luddites or agents of terrorism. The first real indication that this
might not be the case came with the Asian financial collapse in 1997. In the space
of only a few weeks, neoliberal orthodoxy brought over a million people in
Thailand and 22 million in Indonesia below the poverty line.[19] That crisis enabled
millions of people to behold the 'realities.' One of those realities was that the free
world policies imposed by the IMF had not induced in LDCs the levels of growth,
prosperity and equity expected, but rather even greater poverty and inequality.
Can anyone seriously deny that the disastrously bestial attack on the World Trade
Centre in New York on 11 September 2001 had no connection to any of this?

Abroad, the friendly image of neoliberal, 'can-do', freedom-loving American go-
getting came crashing down in a welter of debt and doubt. At home, safe in the
USA itself, the contradictions of global capitalism – deregulated and profit-driven –
obliterated US$ 4.6 trillion of investor wealth. This inaugurated a period of rising
unemployment and economic insecurity from which many Americans still suffer.
Domestically this has resulted in two separate counter-movements – the fight for
social justice, and a militant opposition to the wars in Iraq and Afghanistan.
Abroad, imperial military interventions seemed to dominate, but these generated
opposition, as in South Africa, where the ANC came into power under Nelson
Mandela. Likewise, in the Palestinian Territories, the First Intifada prevented defeat
by US-backed Israel and Lebanon from which the USA finally fled in 1983 after 241
of their marines were killed. Somalia, too, saw President Clinton forced to end US
military intervention in 1993.

The link between neoliberalism and war is becoming increasingly obvious, and
the longer the conflict in Afghanistan and Iraq goes on, the more people recognise this. Perhaps if the war had been quick and decisive, it might not have
attracted such widespread criticism, and might not have caused neoliberalism to
be seen as so closely linked to it. However, in particular, these features of the warfare state of the USA and the UK have effectively shaken the legitimacy of neoliberalism as harbouring any prospects for global equity. Also, it is interesting to
note that none of these three are hugely significant in either military or financial

terms, but they are in moral terms, and it is in the moral context that both an initial concern for global health rights and justice in bringing them about must play the dominant role. There is nothing theoretical about this. It is no longer so much a question of whether the wealthy nations of the world can actually wage a military conflict against 'terrorism', but of when they will realise that this is an impossibility.

One does not need to be an old-style anarchist, or a new-style communist, or indeed an '-ist' of any kind, to recognise that we have to rethink the whole ball game, making human rights an a-priori rather than a 'desirable by-product' of our methodology. Areas of the world that have been particularly egregiously affected by neoliberalism are, not unnaturally, paramount in showing both that it doesn't work globally and long term, and also how to find alternative approaches.

Latin America provides a good example of this. In the past it has kept throwing up opposition movements, many of which were stifled by the ruling juntas in the individual countries affected, backed up by US governments and business interests. However, some have survived these initial setbacks for long enough to establish a tradition on which others can be built. In recent years there have been popular uprisings in Peru, Ecuador, Argentina and Bolivia, and elections in Brazil, Venezuela, Uruguay and Chile that have brought to power political forces that do not regard neoliberalism as the answer. Lula de Silva, Hugo Chavez, Tabaré Vasquez, Evo Morales and Michelle Bachelet differ widely from one another in their ideological perspectives. However, on the basis that each is committed to domestic and international policies that place human rights high on their priority list, they can now cooperate to prevent economic subjugation of the region by free trade policies imposed through the WTO.

Sources of inspiration

Over the centuries we have always faced the question of how to survive both as a species and as individuals in a world full of uncertainty. Of course, every other living creature faces the same problem, but we are unique, as Herodotus pointed out in his *Histories* about 2,500 years ago, in that we can be guided by the memories of other people.[20] The human capacity to share ideas and stories, and above all to write them down for the benefit of future generations, has conferred on us a level of control over our own continued survival that is unique in the animal kingdom.

We have celebrated it in a panoply of art, music, drama, storytelling, religious beliefs, moral codes and various forms of government down the centuries. We are aware of the (comparatively) short lifespan that any one individual has, and thus, as individuals, we typically are in a furious rush to learn as much as possible about how to survive. Of course nothing much can save us if, say, the earth is hit by a huge meteor. However, most disasters with which we have become familiar over the millennia have been ones in which we play some role – either by reacting injudiciously to some natural disaster, or by causing a disaster by our own actions. Attempts to address the latter by developing moral codes and moral sensibilities have been crucial in this endeavour.

Our present predicament with regard to both the environmental crisis and global equity brings us, possibly for the first time in our collective history, face to face with truly important decisions. WH Auden[21] put one of these concerns rather bluntly when he observed that 'We must love one another, or die' in addressing the issue of war. The growing conflict between human lifestyles and the environment makes the same point more forcefully.

We are fortunate in that we are so richly endowed with sources of inspiration for equipping ourselves for the task. There are certainly no reasons at all for believing that the very best system we can come up with is one that guarantees the perpetuation of marginalisation, exploitation, exposure to pandemics, warfare and fear. We can do better than that, but we must move fast because time is running out. To shift the goal of global equity with regard to health (on which all other human rights depend) out of the realm of a pious dream to actual realisation, we need to make radical changes towards internationalism and the elimination of war as a way of resolving political and economic differences. The only existing body that has any realistic hope of now meeting our needs in that respect is the United Nations.

The problem of transnational mediation

The difficulties, already alluded to, in mediating global human rights centre on the seemingly simple idea of some kind of 'world referee' and, moreover, one with the power to adjust global conflicts satisfactorily. The establishment of the League of Nations (1920–1946) seemed to be one way of establishing such a global arbiter. However, that failed. It was succeeded, after the Second World War, by the UN. The latter has been far more successful than the League in establishing global agencies such as the WHO, UNESCO, UNDP, etc., in defining and protecting human rights, and in actually moderating the influence of disastrous situations on the ground. However, in recent years it seems to have become hopelessly mired in such important issues as being able to intervene in order to prevent war, or to protect many of the gains that it has already made.

That the world needs an effective global mediating instrument of some kind is beyond question. But what are the obstacles to the UN, as currently constituted, in fulfilling that role? One obvious stumbling block is the modern concept of 'nation', which has been with us since 1648 (Peace of Westphalia), so it is rather presumptuous of the author to think that a few pages of discourse will resolve the issue! However, the problems that we face are too important for us not to make the attempt. The basic problem of the 'nation' as designated by the Westphalia Treaty is that the nation has 'sovereignty rights' which prevent outside interference with what is going on within its borders, provided that these events are approved by the nation's government. The modern UN has resolved this problem by making exceptions for situations in which a sovereign government is practising 'genocide.' However, the legal definition of 'genocide' is such that discussion about whether or not whatever outrage is being perpetuated constitutes genocide can prevent real remediating action from taking place. A current example is provided by the fate of the people of Darfur under the government of Sudan.

As far back as early 2005 it was clear, and was amply demonstrated by any number of news agencies and independent observers, that the people of Darfur were being systematically attacked and brutalised by forces armed and equipped by the Sudan government. The question of whether what was happening constituted 'genocide' has so far effectively prevented the UN from even imposing trade restrictions on Sudan, let alone sending in peace-keeping forces in large enough numbers to actually make a difference. This is because the UN itself cannot violate national sovereignty. However, even the presence of peace-keeping forces is not always much of a guarantee of human rights, as has been borne out terribly by events in Bosnia and Rwanda just in the last few years.

The example that most graphically demonstrates the contradictions, and over a very long period of time, is undoubtedly the Israeli–Palestinian conflict. Israel has been a nation since 1948, whereas the Palestinian Authority has not yet been so designated. The actual conflict between these two Semitic peoples extends far back into recorded history, and the deals by which the state of Israel came into existence are mired in a sordid history of British, American and other political intrigue. However, although the Palestinian people by and large would welcome a UN peace-keeping force to arbitrate the rights of both groups, this has been consistently disallowed by the Israelis – and Israel is a nation.

Things in that part of the world are, indeed, taking a curious twist as I write these words in July 2006. Israel is currently engaged in military conflict with two of its neighbours – the Palestinian Authority on its west and south-western borders, and the Hezbollah in Lebanon on its northern border. Although it has long resisted any idea of UN peace-keeping forces entering its border zones with the Palestinians, it is now actively seeking such forces in its border zones with Lebanon!

The resolution of this conflict is crucial, not only to peace and human rights in the Middle East, but also globally, because of the US policy of support for Israel. The area is virtually a tinderbox because if Iran and Syria (both of which actively support Hezbollah) become involved, it will have serious international impacts, not least by seriously compromising oil supplies. If one had to put the problem in a sound-bite, it could be this: *the UN is constituted to protect the rights of nations, but not the rights of people.* It has, as already mentioned, set up extremely successful agencies – such as the WHO – which have the protection of human rights as the basis of their mandate – but as an organisation it cannot positively intervene to defend human rights except in very special circumstances. Even the WHO is now restricted in defending the human right to health from the actions of US-based corporate ventures in the LDCs by not being able to overrule the WTO. In other words, the UN has fathered agencies with conflicting mandates on the basic human rights in its own original Charter.

One could indicate all kinds of other difficulties with the UN's capacity to defend and protect the human rights that it promotes so well – for instance, the restricting of the power of veto to only a few very powerful nations. One solution to this could be that some kind of ratio (not 50%, but something like 80%) of Security Council votes could determine UN action. Another problem is that UN peace-keeping forces are often rendered ineffective by restrictions placed on how and when they can intervene. This became very obvious in, for example, both Bosnia in Europe, and Rwanda in Africa.

Another important criterion that a transnational mediating authority would surely have to meet is not only to be able to call up a military force quickly in response to emergencies requiring it, but a force responsible to the command of that authority alone. One obvious way in which this could be done is for the 'World Body', whatever it might be called, to be able to call on different nations for given numbers and types of troops from their regular standing forces. This would allow the World Body to ensure that troops being used to mediate a dispute in, say, countries X and Y, are not drawn from close allies of either country. The present UN might well be modified to meet such a role, but is the phrase 'United Nations' itself meaningful? This author is of the view that whatever we call the World Body, it should not allow its Secretary General ever to say that its first responsibility is to the world's existing states rather than to its peoples! However, even at that, more than a cosmetic change would be required.

Another question that arises concerns what the role of existing nations would be in a world in which a World Body existed as an internationally recognised arbitrator/enforcer. If we ever do end up with a world government as such, it is such a remote and unlikely prospect in this author's view that debate about it cannot realistically be regarded as a solution to our present pressing problems. The issue of human rights itself suggests that some things, by their very nature, transcend the perceived temporary needs of any state's powers. Such rights include the obvious – health, access to primary healthcare, education, freedom from arbitrary arrest or imprisonment, etc. These rights can be safeguarded within the context of a nation state, provided that the nation states themselves are not being made victims, say, through the global free trade rules of other nation states.

For instance, the globalisation of trade is a good idea, but it is probably best implemented by some system of regional fair trade, or equity trade, within clusters of nations. The idea would be to prevent groups of small nations from competing with one another in a race to the bottom in exporting the same commodity (e.g. coffee) to developed nations. The particular clusters do not need to be fixed by statute, but can vary according to the situation. The people refereeing this, in the World Body, would be democratically elected from each nation and decisions would be made by experts in the relevant area as agreed by the elected World Body. For instance, consider the impact on health of infrastructural arrangements for global trade.

Within each nation, there would have to be National Health Impact Assessment as described by the author in a previous book.[22] This would be most effectively mediated within small communities within the nation, but with reference to national codes on health and safety. These national codes would, likewise, have to be consistent with International Health Impact Codes. Before any nation embarked on a system of trade relations with another nation, the World Body would have to first make sure that an International Impact Assessment (IIA) had been made and rules laid down for the infrastructural and other contractual changes required.

None of this would be easy, but we don't really have much choice in the matter, caught as we are between the Charybdis of environmental disaster and the Scylla of such man-made disasters as oil wars caused by neoliberal globalisation. When it comes down to it, we must depend on what can be done and not wait in the hope of some dramatic 'historical inevitability' or, alternatively, that rogue meteor whizzing through space. This author hereby rests his case. We can make the human right to health (and all of the other rights) a possibility and not merely a visionary's dream, but only if we organise on the basis that, although the world's people are marvellously different – singing to different scales, saying the same things in different languages, and having different appearances to each other – the only thing that really matters is our common humanity.

References

1 Elliott L. G8 Progress Report. *The Guardian*, 30 June 2006, p. 13.
2 World Health Organization. *Healthy Life Expectancy.* Geneva: World Health Organization; 2006.
3 UN Development Program. *Human Development Report 2004.* New York: UN Development Program Offices; 2004.
4 AVERT. *AIDS in Africa;* www.avert.org/aids-africa-questions-1.htm (accessed 15 July 2006).
5 US Department of State. *Population Reference Report: Russia's continuing demographic decline.* New York: Columbia University Libraries, Lehman Social Sciences Libraries; 2006.
6 World Health Organization. *The Atlas of Heart Disease and Stroke.* Geneva: World Health Organization; 2006.
7 Mathers C, Loncar D. *Updated Projections of Global Mortality and Burden of Disease from 2002 to 2030.* WHO Policy Working Paper. Geneva: World Health Organization; 2005. pp. 38–41.
8 Global Health 2005. The paths of infections. *Time Magazine.* 2005; **166:** 71–4.
9 World Health Organization. World Health Report 1999. Geneva: World Health Organization; 2000.
10 UNESCO. *MDGs and Health Equity in Cuba.* Human Development Report. Paris: UNESCO; 2005. p. 2.
11 Stiglitz J. *Making Globalisation Work.* Harmondsworth: Penguin Books; 2006. p. 6.
12 Saeed S. *Reserve Currency: will China be able to provide an alternative?* Dawn Internet Edition; www.dawn.com/2003/04/07ebr4.htm (accessed 16 July 2006).
13 Ibid., p. 10.
14 MacDonald T. *Third World Health: hostage to First World wealth.* Oxford: Radcliffe Publishing; 2005. pp. 53–5.
15 Samuelson R. Capitalism in retreat. *Business Week*, 14 September 1998, p. 21.
16 MacDonald T. *Health, Trade and Human Rights.* Oxford: Radcliffe Publishing; 1998. pp. 26–7.
17 Porritt J. *Capitalism as if the World Matters.* London: Earthscan; 2006.
18 Stecopoulos H. *Neoliberal Culture and the United States.* www.cfp.english.upenn.edu/archive/2001-08/0041-html (accessed 19 January 2007).
19 Karunatilleka E. *The Asian Economic Crisis.* Paper written for the UK House of Commons by the Parliamentary Librarian; 1999. www.parliament.uk/commons/lib/research/rp99/rp99-014.pdf (accessed 19 January 2007)
20 Herodotus. *The Histories* (Rawlinson G, translator, Bowder H, editor). London: Everyman, JM Dent; 1992. p. 5.
21 Auden WH. 'September 1, 1939.' In: Williams O, editor. *A Little Treasury of Modern Poetry.* London: Routledge Kegan-Paul; 1940. p. 197.
22 MacDonald T, op. cit., 2005 pp. 221–2.

Endnote

[a] This terrible possibility has been well documented, and out of 30 sources that I have to hand, I cite three:

- www.truthout.org.docus. See *Los Angeles Times* writer Paul Richter's report dated 25 January 2003, entitled 'US weighs tactical nuclear strike in Iraq.'
- www.globalresearch.ca/articles. They have a wealth of material, including some excellent articles by Professor Michael Chossudovsky.
- www.newyorker.com/fact. See Seymore Hersh's article on 'Analysis of National Security', dated 17 April 2006.

Index